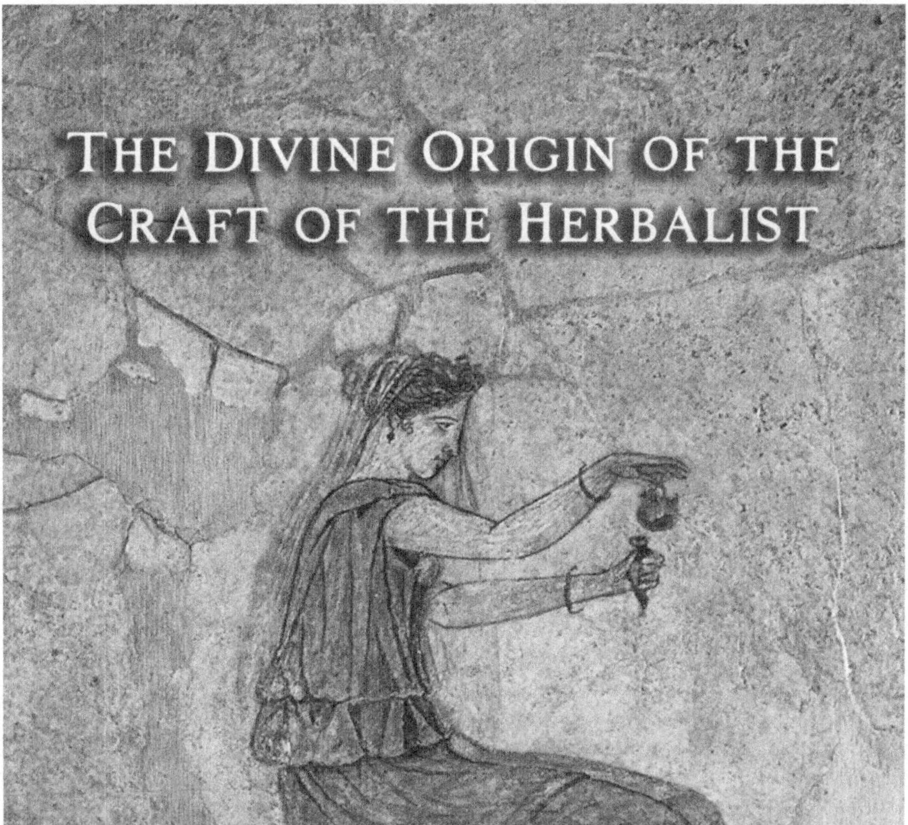
THE DIVINE ORIGIN OF THE
CRAFT OF THE HERBALIST
E.A. WALLIS BUDGE

The Divine Origin of the Craft of the Herbalist
E. A. Wallis Budge

A Cornerstone Book
Published by Cornerstone Book Publishers
An Imprint of Michael Poll Publishing

Cornerstone Book Publishers
New Orleans, LA

This is a photographic reproduction of the 1920 edition of this work.

First Cornerstone Edition - 2013
www.cornerstonepublishers.com

ISBN: 1613421222
ISBN-13: 978-1-61342-122-2

MADE IN THE USA

PREFATORY NOTE

The herb-doctors and physicians of Sumer, Babylon, Assyria and Egypt have proclaimed with no uncertain voice that their craft was founded by the gods, who taught men the curative properties of water, herbs and plants and oils, and who were themselves the first practitioners. And for the last 5000 years men in every civilized country have regarded the divine art of healing as the greatest of the gods' gifts to men. The divine art was carefully and jealously guarded by its recipients, and for many generations was preserved by means of oral tradition. As soon as men learned to write they committed the teaching to the clay tablet and the roll of papyrus, and drew up lists of medicinal herbs, and these documents constituted the first Herbals. The British Pharmacopœia of the present day contains much that is derived from the early Oriental Herbals.

It would be foolish to blink the fact that in ancient Herbals medicine and magic are almost inextricably mixed together; but the broad fact remains, and it is admitted by all competent authorities, that the compilers of the oldest Oriental Lists of Plants and Herbals had a very real knowledge of primitive medicine. But for the ingrained and invincible love of magic in their patients that knowledge would have been greater. From this real knowledge the modern science of herbalism has been developed, just as astronomy owes its origin to Sumerian and Babylonian astrology, and chemistry to alchemy, *i.e.* "the art of Egypt" (*Al*, the Arabic article, *Χημεία*),—or "the art of the land of black earth" (*Χημία*).

The Edwin Smith Papyrus affords evidence that in Egypt at least there were as early as B.C. 2000 herb-doctors and physicians who discarded magic from their treatment of patients, and who understood that sicknesses and diseases were the effects, not of the operations of devils, but of purely natural causes. They practised dissection, and tried to find what these causes were, and the passages of the papyrus already published certainly suggest that such men were genuine seekers after truth, who were as much interested in informing themselves as in helping their patients.

The Asu, or Oriental prototype of the physician, whether Babylonian or Egyptian, of to-day wore a long woollen cloak, and a head cloth in folds, and sandals; when he set out on his rounds he probably rode a donkey. As a herbalist he took with him his box of medicines, and as a magician his wonder-working rod, which was the symbol of his profession. This last was a very important object, and its use among magicians was general. With the rod which was endowed with the power of turning into a serpent, and which God had given to him (Exod. iv. 17), Moses divided the waters of the Sea of Reeds (Exod. iv. 21), and defeated Amalek (Exod. xvii. 11), and brought water out of the rock. And Aaron with his rod turned the waters of the Nile into blood, and produced the plague of frogs (Exod. vii. 19; viii. 6).

The Sumerian herbalist was accompanied by two men, one to recite incantations over the patient (the exorcist), and the other to interpret the omens derived from his condition. The herbalist was the least important of the three, for the divine art of the herb-doctor, strange though it seems, was at that time in thrall to magic, and the herb-doctor himself was subordinate to the exorcist and the interpreter of omens. To-day the physician visits his patients by motor-car, without enchanter and without a reader of omens, for he and his craft are now freed from the bonds of magic. Armed with the true science of medicine, he takes no wonder-working rod with him. But he and his colleagues, like their great predecessor Æsculapius, preserve the memory of and pay honour to the serpent-encircled rod of the Sumerian god Nin̈gishzida, the son of Ninazu, the Master-physician, by making it the symbol of their great profession.

During the past forty years a great deal has been discovered about the forms and contents of Oriental Herbals, but the information given about them in the ordinary text-books is meagre and incomplete. And during the long period when I was Keeper of Egyptian and Assyrian Antiquities in the British Museum I was often called upon to supplement it. I have, therefore, at the request of my friends in the Society of Herbalists, written the following pages on the earliest Oriental Herbals strictly, of course, from the point of view of the archæologist, and described briefly the attributes and works of the earliest gods of medicine in Mesopotamia and Egypt. I have tried to show how the Sumerian, Egyptian, Babylonian and Assyrian Herbals formed the foundation of the Greek Herbals, and how these in turn were translated into Syriac and Arabic and so became known throughout Western Asia, and, thanks to the Nestorian missionary doctors, in Turkestan and China also. For information about the transmission of the Herbals of Dioscorides and Galen into Europe by means of translations into Latin, Italian, German, French, Spanish, Anglo-Saxon, etc., the reader must consult the usual medical Bibliographies. The literary history of the English Herbal has been treated in a competent manner by Miss Eleanour Sinclair Rohde in her *Old English Herbals*, London, 1922, and by Mrs. C. F. Leyel in her admirable book *The Magic of Herbs*, London, 1926.

The illustrations have been made from photographs of manuscripts in the British Museum by permission of the Trustees. The drawing of the serpent-encircled staff, which is, no doubt, the original of the serpent-encircled staves of Æsculapius and Hygieia, is reproduced from Heuzey, *Catalogue des Antiquités Chaldéennes*, Paris, 1902, p. 280. The vase of Gudea, whence the whole scene is taken, is published in De Sarzec, *Découvertes*, Pl. 43, fig. 2.

E. A. WALLIS BUDGE.

48 *Bloomsbury Street,*
Bedford Square,
London, W.C. 1.
November 23, 1927.

CONTENTS

LIST OF ILLUSTRATIONS

"And the Lord God planted a garden eastward in Eden."
GEN. ii. 8.

"The Lord hath created medicines out of the earth."
ECCLUS. xxxviii. 4.

"He causeth herbs to grow for the service of man."
PSALM civ. 14.

"Then give place to the healer, the Lord created him."
ECCLUS. xxxviii. 12.

THE DIVINE ORIGIN OF THE CRAFT OF THE HERBALIST

I

THE OLD GODS AS HERBALISTS AND THEIR DIVINE MEDICINES

THE religious and magical writings of the great nations of antiquity, that is to say, the Chinese and the Indians, the Sumerians and Babylonians, the Persians and Assyrians (or, as we may now call them, the Akkadians), and the Egyptians and Nubians, contain abundant evidence that these primitive peoples believed that the first beings who possessed a knowledge of plants and their healing properties were the gods themselves. They further thought that the substances of plants were parts and parcels of the substances of which the persons of the gods were composed, and that the juices of plants were exudations or effluxes from them likewise. Some of the ancients thought that certain curative plants and herbs contained portions of the souls or spirits of the gods and spirits that were benevolent to man, and that poisonous plants were the abodes of evil spirits that were hostile to the Creator—inasmuch as they destroyed His handiwork, man—and to man and beast.

The oldest gods were too remote from the trivial affairs of the daily life of men to prevent accidents and calamities from overtaking them, but they placed in the hands of their vicars upon earth a certain kind of knowledge and power which, if rightly used, would enable them to annul and destroy the machinations of evil spirits, and bring to nought the works effected by them, and even to alter the courses of natural phenomena in heaven and upon earth. To this knowledge and power the unsatisfactory name of "Magic" has been given, and though primarily the word "Magic" only described the learning of the priests and sages of the Medes and Persians, who were famed for their skill in working enchantments, the word is now used to describe any supposed supernatural art, but more particularly any system of learning or art which claims to control the actions of spiritual or superhuman beings. "Magic" has always appealed greatly to men of all nations, for by the use of it a man ceases to be a supplicant of the gods, and is able to command and to force supernatural beings and things to do his will.

When the gods transmitted the knowledge of plants and their medical properties to their priests, they intended that knowledge to be used for the benefit of their worshippers, whether they were rich or poor, gentle or simple. What the priests had obtained from the gods was not "Magic," or "Natural Magic," but Natural Wisdom, and it was only because those who were treated by the priests did not understand even the rudiments of that wisdom, that they regarded it as "magic" and called it so. As time went on those who applied this natural wisdom to the relief of suffering humanity magnified their office, and introduced into their operations incantations, divinations, astrology and at a later period alchemy. In fact the medical magic of the oldest period represented a confused mass of beliefs and practices which, because they were beyond the ordinary views of cause and effect, were regarded as supernatural. In all ages there have been minds which were not satisfied with the facts and explanations afforded by reason, and these have always served as a fruitful field for the operations of unprincipled priests, and been the dupes of the "magician" and the charlatan.

During the nineteenth century the craft of the herbalist fell into disrepute, chiefly because men's minds were carried away by the discoveries concerning the nature and functions of plants and herbs which were being made by the men who were steadily endeavouring to establish a scientific system of pharmacology. Secondary causes were the intense conservatism and ignorance of the herb-doctors and the dealers in herbs, who refused to believe anything about the world of plants used in medicine which was not to be found in the antiquated Herbals of Grattarola of Bergamo (1515–1568), and Turner's *New Herball*, which was published between 1551 and 1568, and the Herbal of Gerarde (1545–1607), the herb-gardener of Lord Burghley, and the *Physical Directory* which Nicholas Culpeper (born 1616, died 1654) published in 1649. This last-named work in no way deserved the excessive abuse which was heaped upon it by interested persons. Here is an example quoted by the *D.N.B.* from the periodical *Mercurius Pragmaticus*, No. 21, 1649. This book is "done (very filthily) into English by one Nicholas Culpeper, who commenced the several degrees of Independency, Brownisme, Anabaptisme; admitted himself of John Goodwin's schools (of all ungodlinesse) in Coleman Street; after that he turned Seeker,

Manifestarian, and now he is arrived at the battlement of an Atheist, and by two yeeres drunken labour hath Gallimawfred the apothecaries book into nonsense, mixing every receipt therein with some scruples, at least, of rebellion or atheisme besides the danger of poysoning men's bodies. And (to supply his drunkenness and leachery with a thirty shilling reward) endeavoured to bring into obloquy the famous societies of apothecaries and chyrurgeons."

There seems to be little doubt that the *Physical Directory* and Culpeper's later work, the *English Physician Enlarged*, were recognized as authoritative by a very large number of people. Of the last-named work five editions appeared before 1698, and further editions appeared as late as 1802 and 1809. We may note in connection with these facts that Dr. G. A. Gordon prepared a collective edition of Culpeper's works which appeared in 1802.

In these works, and in others of similar character, common sense and even common decency were alike set at nought, and in these days it is very hard to understand how prescriptions like the following could ever have been written and published.

> 1. For Epilepsy.—" Vitriol, calcined until it becomes yellow; saturate with alcohol, add mistletoe, hearts of peonies, elks' hoofs, and the pulverized skull of an executed malefactor (!): distil all these dry, rectify the distillate over castoreum (species diamoschi dulcis), elephants' lice: then digest in a water-bath for a whole month, after mixing with salt of peony, alcohol, liquor salis perlarum et corallorum, oil of anisi and succini " (Baas, *Hist. Med.*, p. 436).

2. Tincture of Mummy.—" Select the cadaver of a red, uninjured, fresh, unspotted malefactor 24 years old, and killed by hanging, broken (*sic*) on the wheel, or impaled, upon which the moon and the sun have shone once: cut it in pieces, sprinkle with myrrh and aloes; then macerate for a few days, pour on spirits," etc. (*Ibid.*, p. 136).

3. Extraction of a Tooth.—" The powder of earthworms, of mice dung, and of a hare's tooth, put into the hole of a rotten tooth, it will drop out without any instrument" (Culpeper's *Last Legacy*, p. 107).

The men who invented and published such disgusting prescriptions as the above did the craft of the herbalist much harm, but it must also be confessed that in the "sixties" and "seventies" of the last century the state of the herbalists' shops, especially those which were situated in the outlying districts of London, was not calculated to increase the faith of the public in the efficacy of herbs, or belief in the knowledge of those who sold them. Many of my contemporaries will remember a herbalist's shop which was situated in a popular street near King's Cross in the year 1865, and its dirty and unkempt appearance. The shop proper was about 8 feet wide and 20 feet long. Its window front was glazed with small panes of bottle-green glass, which were seldom washed or cleaned, and on the brightest day very little light entered the shop through them; during the winter months, and especially in foggy weather, the shopkeeper was obliged to carry on his business by the light of two or three guttering "dips," *i.e.*

tallow candles. A low narrow counter took up much of the floor space. On one end of this stood a rickety glass case containing small bowls of seeds and berries, which were well coated with dust, and on the other stood a pair of rusty iron scales and a huge glass bowl of a mixture called "sarsaparilla wine." Men and women, as well as the children, who came in and spent their halfpennies and pennies freely drank this wine out of teacups of various sizes and shapes and makes, which were rarely rinsed in water, and were usually turned bottom upwards on the counter to dry. A large cardboard label was tied round the bowl, and on this were written in large capitals the names of all the ailments and sicknesses which this particular brand of sarsaparilla wine was said to cure.

On the end wall was a shelf whereon stood a couple of ostrich egg-shells, and several bottles containing "preparations" of various kinds, of a most uninviting appearance, and two human skulls. Below the shelf, nailed to the wall, was a small dried crocodile or lizard, and below this a miscellaneous collection of dried "specimens," all richly coated with dust. To the wall behind the counter several narrow shelves were fastened. On one of these stood a row of yellow glazed pottery jars on which were painted the names of herbs and compounds; some had covers and some had not, and the legends were half concealed by dust. On another shelf was a series of small bottles and flasks which contained extracts, or decoctions, of herbs, medicated unguents and perfumes and vegetable oils. Another shelf was filled with bottles of medicated sweets, such as paregoric drops, squills, lozenges, sticks of horehound candy, "stick liquorice," etc., and these sweets were in great demand by juvenile customers. From the ceiling and on the wall in front of the counter hung bundles of dried herbs, lavender, rosemary, mint, camomile, dandelion, sorrel and many others, all well covered with dust. Under the counter were wooden boxes containing poppy-heads, senna leaves, marsh-mallow, linseed meal, etc., and a stock of paper bags and phials of various sizes.

The proprietor sold his wares rather by "rule of thumb" than by measures or scales, and he eschewed the writing of directions for the use of his patients. He was old and very shabby, but kindly, and many of his customers were evidently friends and acquaintances, judging by the way in which he advised them as to their ailments. His shop was well patronized by children, who came there to see him exhibit "Pharaoh's serpents." He would set on a plate a lump of some brown substance rather like chocolate, and when he applied a lighted match to a certain part of it, the lump changed its shape and heaved, and from its sides several spirals emerged and went wriggling across the plate like worms, to the great delight of the onlookers. When asked why these wriggling things were called "Pharaoh's serpents," he said that he did not know, but that his father and his grandfather had always called them by this name. When he was unable to advise a customer, he used to knock the counter with a weight, and then his wife, a little old wizened woman, would appear from behind the shop and take charge of the case. It was generally thought that she was the real herbalist to the establishment, and certainly her reputation in the neighbourhood was great.

The shop described above and its contemporary herbal establishments have long since passed away, and the modern establishments of the Society of Herbalists leave nothing to be desired. There are now many signs that the craft of the herbalist in Great Britain is regaining its rightful position among the systems of medicine which have been evolved by the generations of men in their efforts to heal the sicknesses and diseases which attack their bodies and which, if not annulled, destroy life itself. For the general public have learned that the methods now used in extracting the essential juices, etc., from medicinal herbs, and in the preparation of extracts, tinctures, etc., are scientific and accurate. Moreover the effects of herbal drugs on the body are better known and understood, and it is now possible to obtain herbal preparations of uniform strength and quality.

II

THE DIVINE HERBALISTS

It has already been said that many ancient nations thought that the gods themselves were the first herbalists, and that it was they who had taught their vicars upon earth how to heal the sicknesses of mankind by means of certain herbs and plants. More than this, they thought that the herbs and plants which the gods employed in their work of healing were composed of or contained parts of the bodies of the gods. And as the operation or effect of a medicine became more assured, or more potent, if a formula was recited at the time when it was administered to the patient, the god or goddess supplied, according to the general belief, the words which constituted the formula which was recited by the herbalist. Thus the medicine itself, and the knowledge of how to administer it, and its healing effect, came directly from the gods. It is then clear that the gods were the earliest herbalists and physicians.

It is impossible to say exactly which nation possessed the oldest gods of medicine. Of the Chinese gods of medicine little seems to be known. Some authorities claim that an Emperor of China called Huang-ti, who reigned about B.C. 2637, composed a treatise on medicine, and that another emperor, Chin-nong (B.C. 2699), composed a catalogue of Chinese herbs, or a sort of pharmacopœia, but satisfactory evidence in support of these statements is wanting.

We have it on the high authority of Dr. Lionel Barnett that the early history of Indian medicine is very obscure. That very ancient work the Athara-vēda contains a vast quantity of spells to heal sickness, exorcise demons, and overpower sorcerers, love-charms (as a rule by no means innocent), and incantations of various kinds. None of the works in use in the medical schools of India is older than the beginning of the Christian era, and we cannot, therefore, consider the gods of India as the oldest herbalists or physicians.

Many Greek writers describe the remarkable skill of the Egyptian physicians, and refer to the great antiquity of the study of medicine in Egypt, and it was thought for a very long time that the dwellers on the Nile were the inventors of the art of healing. Manetho tells us (Cory's *Fragments*, p. 112) that Athōthis, the son of Mēnes, the second king of the Ist Dynasty, was a physician, and that he left behind him books on anatomy. Now the latest date we can give to this king is about B.C. 3600, but Nārmer-Men, whom the Greeks knew as Mēnes, was a foreigner, and there is reason to believe that he came from some country to the east of Egypt. Therefore the books on anatomy which his son, or grandson, left behind him, were probably works by men who were not Egyptians.

The tombs and the buildings of the successors of Athōthis prove that in their time the arts and crafts had attained a high pitch of perfection, and certain chapters of the *Book of the Dead* were either composed or introduced into the official religion at this period. It is difficult to believe that the indigenous

Egyptian did all the things that he is claimed to have done, and more difficult still to think that he built the famous "Step Pyramid" (still 197 feet in height), except at the suggestion of and with the help of foreigners. Imhetep, the Wazîr of King TCHESER, whose tomb the Step Pyramid was intended to be, was a great architect and a great physician, and was worshipped as a god after his death. The Greeks identified him with their great god of medicine, Æsculapius, and Manetho says that he "built a house of hewn stones, and greatly patronized writing." We may note in passing that this house of hewn stones has been recently discovered by Mr. C. Firth of the Egyptian Service of Antiquities, and excavated.

Now it must not be assumed that the indigenous Egyptians had no knowledge of the use of herbs in medicine in the fourth millennium B.C.; on the contrary, there is reason to believe that they were well acquainted with most of the herbs and plants which we find mentioned in the great Ebers Papyrus. But it is very probable that the medical knowledge of their Asiatic conquerors was greater than their own, and that Imhetep was the first to reduce to writing or to edit for them an authoritative book of medicine. It is a well-known fact that no satisfactory translation of the Ebers Papyrus has been made, or can be made, for the simple reason that we do not know how to translate the names of scores of herbs and plants which are found in the prescriptions. It is possible that these are the ancient native names of herbs and plants which were well known throughout the Nile Valley, but not to the later dynastic Egyptians.

The principal Egyptian gods and goddesses who were specially skilled in medicine and the art of healing were these: Osiris was a god of vegetation in one of his earliest phases, and at all periods he was associated with the moon. He was skilled in the knowledge of plants and was a great agricultural authority, and he introduced wheat and one kind of barley into Egypt; he taught men the cultivation of the vine and was the first god to make wine. As the god and judge of the dead he dwelt in a portion of the Tuat or Underworld, and the souls of the beatified dead spent their time there in the cultivation of the wonderful *Maat* plant. This plant or shrub was a form of the body of Osiris, and his followers ate it and lived upon it. It maintained their lives, and because they ate the body of their god, they became one with him and, like him, lived for ever.

Closely associated with Osiris was the goddess Isis, his twin sister and wife. Her knowledge of herbs was great, and, as one of the most ancient Mother-goddesses of Egypt, she was the great protectress of her husband Osiris, her son Horus, and women and children in general. In the Ebers Papyrus (Plate I) she is addressed thus: "May Isis heal me as she healed Horus of all the wounds which his brother Set, who slew his father Osiris, had inflicted upon him. O Isis, thou great magician, heal me, and deliver thou me from all bad, evil and Typhonic things, and from every kind of fatal sickness, and from diseases caused by devils, and from impurity of every kind, even as thou didst deliver thy son Horus from such." In the same Papyrus (Plate XLVII) we have a prescription for pains in the head which she wrote for the god Rā. As a woman Isis suffered from some ailment in her breast, and a copy of the prescription for the medicine which she prepared and used herself is given on Plate XCV.

But Isis was a great magician as well as a great herbalist, and by means of the series of invincible spells which she was taught by THOTH, and by the use of the secret name of the Sun-god RĀ, she could vanquish every sorcerer, loose every spell, destroy the effect of all incantations and poisons, and raise the dead. Thus when Osiris was slain by his brother SET, and Isis found his dead body lying on the dyke at Netat near Abydos in Upper Egypt, she brought it into the city and restored life to it for a season by means of the magical touch of her sex and the powerful spells which she uttered. Osiris rose up from his state of inertness, and consorted with Isis, and their son HORUS was born as a result of this embrace. One day, whilst living in the papyrus swamps of the Delta, she was obliged to leave her son Horus for a short time, and during her absence Set sent a scorpion, which crawled to the place where the child was sleeping and stung him to death. When Isis returned and found his dead body, she appealed to Rā, who stopped the Boat of Millions of Years in which he was sailing over the sky, and sent down Thoth to help her. Thoth imparted to her certain words of power, and when these were uttered by the goddess Horus was restored to life.

On one occasion Isis used her knowledge of poisonous herbs for a selfish purpose. She wished to possess as much power as Rā, and to learn the secret name by virtue of which he ruled the heaven and the earth, and gods and men. As Rā did not wish to reveal his secret name to her, she made a reptile, and having recited enchantments over it, she set it by the side of the road over which Rā travelled daily. As Rā passed the reptile it bit or stung him, and the poison which it injected into the god was so deadly, and so swift in its working, that the strength of the god ebbed rapidly and he was nigh unto death. Isis approached the god as he was in his death agony, and promised him that if he would reveal his secret name to her she would heal him. In his extremity Rā did so, and as the result of the incantations which Isis pronounced forthwith the god recovered.

The god THOTH, to whom Isis appealed in her distress, was himself a very great and powerful physician and magician, and was the author of all the formulas which enabled human physicians to heal sicknesses and to drive out devils and evil spirits from the bodies of their patients. His name was so powerful that if a man called himself Thoth, he at once acquired the attributes of the god. Thoth had on certain occasions practised as a physician, for he treated the Eye of Horus, *i.e.* the Sun, when it was wounded by Set, and restored it to its normal condition. During the fight between Horus and Set, Thoth seems to have had his arm either broken or seriously injured, and he was obliged to employ his knowledge of medicine and magic to heal himself. On another occasion he was associated with Rā in composing a prescription for catarrh in the nose, or perhaps a kind of influenza (Ebers Papyrus, Plate XC). From the earliest times Thoth was regarded as the author and copyist of the powerful spells which he used, and he possessed in a very full degree that marvellous quality or power called HEKA, which Rā himself had invented for the benefit of gods and

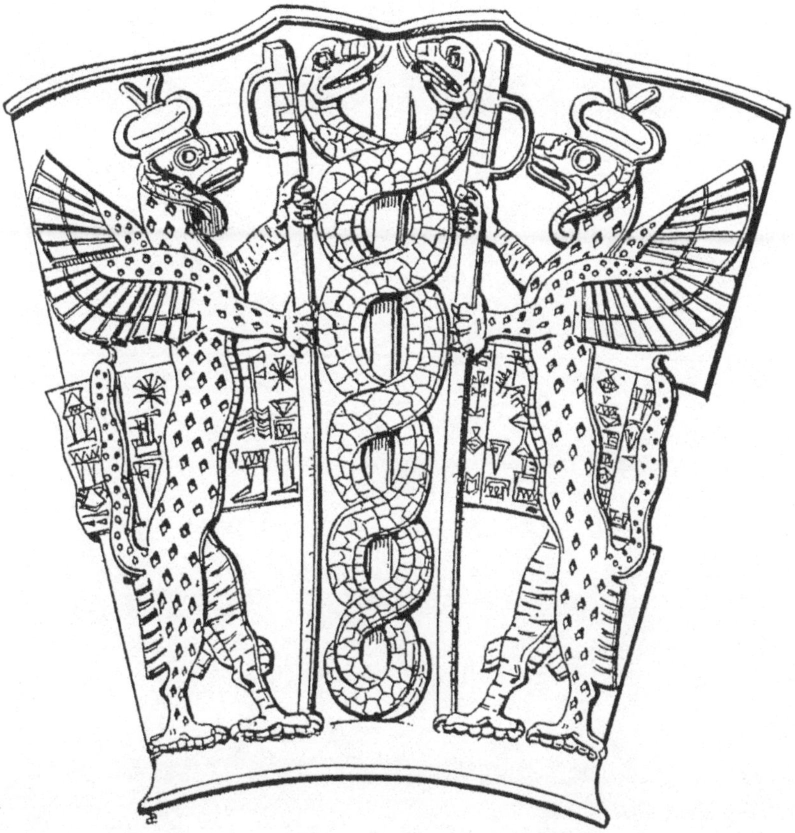

In the centre is a staff with two serpents twined about it, the emblem of the Sumerian god Ningishzida, the son of Ninazu, the Master-physician. On each side is a fabulous composite creature wearing a headdress with horns, and having the head, wings and claws of an eagle and a serpent tail; each holds a staff. The names and attributes and functions of these mythological creatures are not known.

(From a vase dedicated to the god by Gudea, King of Babylonia, B.C. 2350.)

men. He was at once the heart or tongue of Rā, and the secretary of Rā, and as the Keeper of the Book of the god he bore the title of KHER HEB. In late dynastic times he was called "Thoth the thrice great," or "Thoth the thrice greatest," and in bas-reliefs the Thoth of Nubia is represented as holding the *ānkh* or symbol of life in his left hand, and in his right a staff round which a serpent is coiled. We may note in connection with this serpent-encircled staff, that the symbol of the Sumerian god Ningishzida, the son of Ninazu, was a staff around which two serpents were coiled. The serpent was chosen as a symbol of renewed life or immortality because it sloughed its skin, and so apparently renewed its life and health. As already stated, the serpent-encircled staff is the symbol of physicians to this day.

Another most important god of medicine was ANPU, whom the Greeks called "Anubis." He may be regarded as the Apothecary of the gods of Egypt, for he was the keeper of the house of medicines and the "chamber of embalmment." The dead body of Osiris was taken to him, and whilst Isis recited her spells and incantations, Anubis carried out the operations connected with the embalmment of the body of the god and the preservation of his viscera. The cult of the god in Egypt is very ancient, and the introduction to a prescription in the Ebers Papyrus (Plate CIII) says that the prescription itself was taken from a book which was found under the feet of the god Anubis in the town of Letopolis, and that the book was taken to Semti, the fifth king of the Ist Dynasty. In the medical papyrus at Berlin this book is said to have been taken after the death of King Semti, to Sent, a king of the IInd Dynasty.

Thus it is clear that the Egyptians possessed books of medicine in the first half of the fourth millennium before Christ, and that Anubis was even at that early period regarded as the Apothecary and the maker-up of prescriptions for the gods. Anubis was the keeper of mummies in the Other World, and we see him taking part in the weighing of the heart of the dead in the Hall of Osiris, and examining the tongue of the Great Scales on behalf of Thoth and Osiris. The animal sacred to him was a dog or jackal, and together with Upuatu he conducted the souls of the dead from this world to the kingdom of Osiris. We may note in passing that the Sumerian goddess Gula, "who made the dead to live," the wife of Ninurta, is represented seated on a throne with a dog at her feet. In one of their magical systems the Gnostics connected Christ, as the Saviour and knower of hearts, with Anubis, the embalmer and preserver of the hearts of men.

In the legend of the "Destruction of Mankind" by the goddess Hathor we read that Rā caused 7000 vessels of drugged bees to be made. The drug used for the purpose was *tataiti,* which grew in abundance at Elephantine, at the foot of the First Cataract; Brugsch and others have translated the word by "mandrakes," but this rendering is not generally accepted.

Another great god of medicine was Khonsu, who with Amen and Mut formed the first triad of Thebes. One form or phase of him called Khonsu Nefer-hetep devoted himself to the cure of those who suffered from mental ailments. It is recorded that the Prince of Bekhten sent an envoy to Rameses II (?), King of Egypt, who had married one of the Prince's daughters, asking him to send a physician to Bekhten to heal his youngest daughter, who was grievously sick. Rameses sent a physician to Bekhten, but he was unable to heal the Princess, and the Prince, her father, sent a second time to Rameses, and asked that a god might be sent to heal his daughter. With the consent of Khonsu, the god Khonsu Nefer-hetep was sent, and he found on arrival that the Princess was possessed of a devil. The god easily cast out the devil from the Princess, and restored her to health forthwith. The Prince of Bekhten made a great feast, at which both the god and the devil assisted, and the devil was permitted to depart to his own place. Unfortunately the Egyptian text does not tell us whether spells or medicines were employed by the god in casting out the devil from the Princess.

III

WATER A DIVINE ELEMENT

MAN cannot live by bread alone, although wheat was believed to have been formed of the body of God, and without water he could not live at all. His whole existence depends upon it, and from the earliest times man has regarded water as a thing of mystery and has attributed to it supernatural and animistic powers. It gave life to himself and the beasts and the vegetable creation, and it was to him a thing of indefinable and inscrutable origin, and possessed of a divine essence. According to the Egyptians the oldest thing in the world was the great watery abyss called "NU" or "NENU," and from this sprang the first god, RĀ, or KHEPERA, who created the heavens and the earth from the germs which existed in the abyss. From out of this abyss the primeval god sent a river into Egypt, which was thought to enter the country from two openings in the bases of the rocks at the First Cataract, and this river we know as the Nile. The throne of Osiris was set over or by this river, and when the Egyptians became Christians they placed the throne of God by the great river of heaven, whence came the Nile, and He regulated the supply of water to Egypt with His feet. To the Egyptians water was the "Father of the gods," and the Nile was the "water of life," which not only preserved life in the living but revivified the dead. In Babylonia the great rivers the Tigris and Euphrates had their origin in the great primeval abyss Apsū, which was the abode of the god Ea. As in Egypt, so it was in Babylonia, water was holy and divine, and was, of course, worshipped as a god. Both in Egypt and Babylonia it was used largely in medical, magical and religious ceremonies of all kinds, for it was regarded as the supreme cleanser of both soul and body. Pagan philosophers believed that water was in existence before God created the heavens and the earth, and the Egyptian Christians said, "there is no one whatsoever who knoweth anything about the creation of water except God Himself." They also placed water, the wheat plant and the throne of the Father in one category, and regarded them as the equivalents of the Son of God. In scores of prescriptions given in the Ebers Papyrus water forms one of the principal ingredients of the medicines.

As to the wheat plant. From the Egyptian texts we know that in one of his many aspects, or phases, Osiris was a grain-god, and Greek writers say that he introduced wheat and the vine into Egypt and many other countries. Egyptian texts and pictures indicate that wheat plants were believed to spring from his body, and the grains of wheat were parts of it. The Egyptian Christians adopted this view, only they substituted the body of God for the body of Osiris, as we see from the following legend:—Adam and Eve being expelled from Paradise, where they had lived upon choice food, were unable to eat the coarser foods which they found outside Paradise, and in consequence they suffered greatly from hunger and want, and were nigh to die of starvation. Our Lord, Who was Adam's sponsor, went to the Father and asked Him if He wished Adam, whom He had created in His own image, to die of starvation. In answer the Father told our Lord that He had better give His own flesh to Adam to eat, and He did so. Our Lord took flesh from His right side and rubbed it down into grains, and took it to the Father, Who, on seeing that our Lord had obeyed His command, took some of His own flesh, which was invisible, and formed it into a grain of wheat, and placed it with the flesh of His Son. He then sealed the grain of wheat in the middle with the " seal of light," and told our Lord to take the grain and give it to Michael the Archangel, who was to take it to Adam on earth and teach him how to sow and reap it, and how to make bread. When Michael came to Adam he found him by the Jordan and learned from him that he had had nothing to eat for eight days. This legend is found in a Coptic manuscript in the British Museum (Orient. No. 7026). The Coptic text is published with an English translation by Budge, *Coptic Apocrypha*, London, 1913, p. 59 f. and p. 241 f. In an Assyrian text published by R. C. Thompson we find Shamash, the Sun-god, and Sin, the Moon-god, associated with the growing of wheat. Thus we read : " Thou didst make the standing crop to spring up : reaping, binding; binding, ear; ear, [threshing ?]. Shamash when he reaped, Sin when he garnered . . ." (*Proc. Royal Society of Medicine*, 1924, Vol. XVII. pp. 1–34). The prescriptions in the Ebers Papyrus show that flour, dough, and bread, fresh or stale or toasted, were all used in medicine as valuable ingredients.

Returning for a moment to the belief in the holiness of water, we may refer to the water of the ancient and famous Sun-well at Heliopolis. The pagan

Egyptians attached great importance to bathing in the water of this well, and believed that purity of soul and health of body were obtained by the bather thereby. The reason for this belief was the ancient Egyptian tradition that when Rā, the Sun-god, rose on the world for the first time he bathed his face in the water of that well. According to Christian tradition, Mary washed our Lord in water drawn from this well, and when the water was thrown out on the ground, wherever any drops of it fell, balsam trees sprang up. From these shrubs a "holy oil" called "Mērōn" was expressed, which was used for anointing at baptisms and consecrations and other important sacred rites and ceremonies. For centuries it was used as the oil of consecration *par excellence*, and when, as it sometimes happened, a supply of it was not forthcoming, consecrations of ecclesiastical officials had to be postponed.

IV

VEGETABLE SUBSTANCES OF DIVINE ORIGIN

According to a magical papyrus in the British Museum (No. 10051, Salt 825), the connection between the gods and certain vegetable substances was very close. The tears that fall from the eyes of Horus turn into the gum *ānti*, i.e. myrrh. The blood that falls from the nose of Gebban turns into cedar trees, the sap of which is the oil "Sefi." On certain occasions Shu and Tefnut weep, and when their tears reach the ground they sink into the earth and transform themselves into the plants from which incense is made. When Rā weeps copiously the water on falling on the ground becomes "the flies that build," *i.e.* bees, and these, working in the flowers in every garden, produce honey and wax. The Water Flood (*i.e.* the annual Inundation of the Nile) on earth is composed of the sweat which falls from Rā when he is weary, and the other exudations from him turn into papyrus plants. The sweat of the goddesses Isis and Nephthys turns into plants. Rā in the house of the Sun-stone sweats, Ptah in Tanen sweats, Khnemu in the Qerti of Elephantine sweats, Osiris in Tetu sweats, and Shu and Tefnut collect these sweats and fashion them into plants that are the members of the god. The blood of Osiris became the Nārt tree of Amentt, and the blood of Set became the Nārt tree of Abydos. All the plants and the oils of the trees mentioned above were believed to be powerful medicines, and played very important parts in all the rites and ceremonies connected with the resurrection of the dead. In the Græco-Roman period children and others were buried in pots filled with honey, and the body of Alexander the Great is said to have been preserved in " white honey which had not been melted."

V

ANCIENT EGYPTIAN HERBALS AND BOOKS OF MEDICINE

THOUGH there is good reason for believing that official Schools of Herbalists existed in Egypt as early as B.C. 3000, not one of the theoretical works on which the physicians of that day based their practice has come down to us. All the copies of medical papyri now known [1] were written after B.C. 1800, and their contents are series of prescriptions which were probably in general use among the various schools of herbalists in the country. The actual prescription is preceded by a description of the symptoms of the disease which the medicine is intended to cure, and is followed by instructions for the preparation of the ingredients, and for the taking of the medicine by the patient. In some cases a magical formula, which is to be recited sometimes by the physician and sometimes by the patient, is added. It is possible that the libraries in the temples, or those of private individual physicians, contained books dealing with

[1] These are :—(1) the great Ebers Papyrus (published in facsimile with a glossary by Stern at Leipzig, in 1875; transcript by Wreszinski, Leipzig, 1913). (2) The great medical papyrus at Berlin (No. 3032, published by Brugsch and Wreszinski). (3) The medical papyrus in the British Museum (No. 10059). (4) The Hearst Papyrus (published by Wreszinski in 1912). (5) The Kahun Papyrus, published by Griffith. (6) The Edwin Smith Papyrus (described at some length in *Recueil d'Études Égyptologiques*, Paris, 1922, p. 386 ff.).

the theory of medicine, and complete lists of plants or Herbals, but nothing of the kind is known to exist at the present time. The prescriptions show that the Egyptians used animals and animal products, and mineral substances, as well as plants in their medicines, but there is no doubt that five-sixths of the ingredients were of vegetable origin. We find as ingredients in prescriptions the dung of asses, dogs, pigs, gazelle, crocodile, etc., and many other evil-smelling and evil-tasting stuffs such as rotten fish and the gall of various animals; but this need not surprise us, for we find the very same substances are prescribed in Babylonian, Greek, Syrian and European Herbals.

The men who cut open and prepared the bodies of the dead for mummification by removing the viscera and brains, must have known something of elementary surgery, but it seems clear from the material now available that neither they nor the physicians possessed any real knowledge of Anatomy and Physiology. Yet the Egyptians were renowned in ancient days for their knowledge of plants and herbs, and Hippocrates and others incorporated in their writings many prescriptions which they had taken from the medical papyri of the Egyptians. There may have been, and there probably were, many physicians and herbalists who studied plants and anatomy in a scientific manner, and who tried to understand the working of the organs of the body, and the actual effect of the herbal medicines which they prescribed for their patients. Such men, if they existed, no doubt made experiments and noted the results which they obtained; and it is probable that some physicians endeavoured to discover Nature's operations by means of dissection and even by vivisection. But the majority of practitioners relied upon the use of spells and magical ceremonies, and made their treatment to suit the views of their patients, who as a whole believed in magic. The progress of herbal science was strangled by the belief in magic which was general among the people. Men thought that every illness was caused by the operation of one devil, or more than one, who had occupied the limb or member of the body, and had destroyed the protecting influence of the god or good spirit that usually dwelt in it. The first thing to do was to expel the devil, and this could only be effected by a spell or the utterance of the name of some great god; when the devil had been expelled the herbal treatment of the body began. Every member of the body of a living man was protected by a god, and the *Book of the Dead* (Chap. XLII) shows us that the members of a dead man were believed to be protected in the same way. Thus Pepi I, a king of the VIth Dynasty, says: "My hair is Nu. My face is Aten. My eyes are Hathor. My head is Horus. My nose is Thoth. My mouth is Khens-ur. My backbone is Sma. My breast is Babu. My heart is Bastit. My belly is Nut. My phallus is Hapi. My thighs are Nit and Serqit," etc. And in the Papyrus of Nu in the British Museum (No. 10477, sheet 6) the deceased says: "There is no member of my body which is not the member of some god. The god Thoth shieldeth my whole body and I am Rā (the Sun-god) day by day."

VI

HOLY OILS AND MEDICATED UNGUENTS

THE Sumerian, Akkadian and Egyptian herbalists learned at a very early period in their history the value of vegetable oils for the soothing and the healing of the body and the feeding of its tissues. They found that oil protected the skin from the heat of the sun by day, and that it enabled them to endure more easily the bitter cold by night in the deserts of Egypt and the Sūdān and in the bleak plains of Mesopotamia. In Egypt the vegetable oils were thought to be effluxes from the body of Rā, the Sun-god, which had taken the form of certain trees, *e.g.* the olive, the acacia, the palm, etc. Whether the Egyptians thought that the gods and goddesses needed oils for their personal use is not clear, but it is quite certain that in all periods offerings of pure oil and perfumed oil or scented unguent (*Metchet*) were made by worshippers, and were accepted by the gods. Wine was offered at the same time as the oil, and from the antiquity of the custom, which was widespread, we may assume that the gods were supposed to gladden their hearts with the wine and refresh their bodies by anointing them with the oil. The primitive herbalist used oil both to keep the body in health and to nourish it, and, as we see from many prescriptions in the Ebers Papyrus, used it freely in his medicines.

Very soon, however, the anointing of the body came to have a ritual significance, and eventually Unction came to play a very important part in sacramental religion. The dead were anointed as well as the living, and the presence of the oil on their bodies was believed to assist their resurrection. Like water, oil was regarded as a thing of mystery, and a holy character was assigned to it. The HOLY OILS were seven in number and were called Seth-heb, Heknu, Sefth, Nemu, Tuaut, Ha-āsh, Ha-ent-Thehennu. Examples of the anointing tablets on which the names of these oils are inscribed can be seen in the British Museum (Nos. 6122, 6123, 29421). They were used in the tombs of Egypt under the Old Kingdom (about B.C. 2500). At the presentation of each oil the KHER-HEB or priest recited a magical formula or spell, and sometimes he made motions with his professional rod or staff with the view of increasing the effect of the oil on the body. In the Ebers Papyrus several kinds of oil are mentioned, *e.g.* "white oil," "clear oil," "*Aber* oil," "tree oil," "olive oil" (*Baq*). A special oil was used in circumcision (*Tsheps*), and Tchet oil was an ingredient in the famous incense called "Kyphi." The primitive herbalist was the first to discover the value of oil as a medicine, and it was by acting upon his knowledge that the priest was able to turn the secular act into a religious ceremony. The anointed one became holy because a holy substance had been incorporated in him; among the Hebrews anointing was believed to endow the man chosen by them to be their king with the Divine Essence. And Jesus the "Messiah" (*i.e.* "Meshīkhā," the "anointed One," *i.e.* Christos) was endowed with the Holy Ghost.

Another thing realized quickly by the primitive herbalist was that oil was a first-class vehicle in which to administer medicines to the sick; in some of the prescriptions in the Ebers Papyrus we are told to boil all the ingredients together in honey and oil, or in oil alone. He also discovered that men and women were glad to anoint their bodies with *perfumed oils*, and thus originated the trade in ointments, salves, pomades and scented unguents which has assumed such great proportions in our own days. The Ebers Papyrus contains more than a dozen prescriptions for salves and ointments, and the preparation of scented as well as medicated oils and unguents was from the earliest times a very important branch of the herbalist's business.

The perfuming and anointing of the body became at a very early period a part of the RITUAL OF CEREMONIAL DRESS, both of the living and the dead. Jezebel the wife of Ahab (as we read in 2 Kings ix. 30) "set her eyes in paint" and decorated her head before the arrival of Jehu. And one of the mummies found at Dēr al-Baharī shows that the custom of anointing the eyelids of dead princesses, and colouring their lips red, and staining the nails of the fingers and toes reddish-yellow with the juice of the *henna* plant (*Lawsonia inermis*) was prevalent in Egypt. Whether the "lip-stick" was known to the Egyptians is not clear. In a painting on a papyrus at Turin a lady is seen holding a mirror in one hand and colouring her lips with what looks like a reed or pencil which she holds in the other; but this object may well have been the ancient equivalent of the "lip-stick."

One favourite way of applying unguent to the body in use among the Egyptians is made known to us by pictures in the tombs. Men and women alike fastened on the top of the head a sort of conical cage made of some light material like grass, and in this they placed a large lump of scented unguent which touched the hair. The heat of the head melted the unguent, which gradually ran down over the head and saturated the hair and dripped down on to the neck and shoulders. The relatives of the dead placed in the tombs supplies of this unguent, together with metal or alabaster shells on which to prepare it for use. Small bottles and flasks, made of alabaster or glass, filled with scented oils and ointments, were also placed in the tombs, and many hundreds of these may be seen in the British Museum. The Egyptian herbalist paid great attention to the care of the skin, and even provided the dead with pieces of pumice-stone with which to rub down callosities (see the funerary coffer of the lady Anhai in the British Museum).

The herbalist also provided means for preventing baldness. One means was to mix together fat of the lion, fat of the hippopotamus, fat of the crocodile, fat of the cat, fat of the serpent, and fat of the Nubian ibex, and rub the mixture on the head.

The following hair-wash was used for Queen Shesh, the mother of King Teta :—

The claw of a dog, Decayed palm leaves, The hoof of an ass,	in equal quantities.

Boil thoroughly in oil in a pipkin and rub the mixture on the head.

To keep the hair from falling out :—

1. Mix together artists' colour, collyrium, *Khet* plants, oil, gazelle dung and hippopotamus fat, and rub the mixture on the head.

2. Mix crushed flax seed with an equal quantity of oil, add water from a well, and rub the mixture on the head.

3. Boil a lizard in oil and rub the oil on the head. (Ebers Papyrus, Plates LXVI, LXVII.)

As specimens of other prescriptions of the Egyptian herbalist may be quoted :—

1. AGAINST COSTIVENESS. Honey, seeds of raisins, absinth, elder-berries, berries of the *uān* tree, kernels of the *utchāit* fruit, caraway seeds, *āām* seed, *thām* seed and sea-salt in equal quantities; make up into a bolus and administer through the anus. (Ebers Papyrus, Plate IX.)

2. TO STOP DIARRHŒA. Spring onions $\frac{1}{8}$, Groats recently boiled $\frac{1}{8}$, Oil and Honey $\frac{1}{4}$, Wax $\frac{1}{16}$, and $\frac{1}{3}$ of a *tena* of water; boil together and drink for four days. (Ebers Papyrus, Plate XIV.)

3. TO EMPTY THE BELLY and clear out all impurities from the body of a sick person. Field Herbs $\frac{1}{8}$, Honey $\frac{1}{8}$, Dates $\frac{1}{3}$, *uāh* grain; mix together and chew for one day. (Ebers Papyrus, Plate VII.)

The following is a transcript of the hieratic text in hieroglyphs :

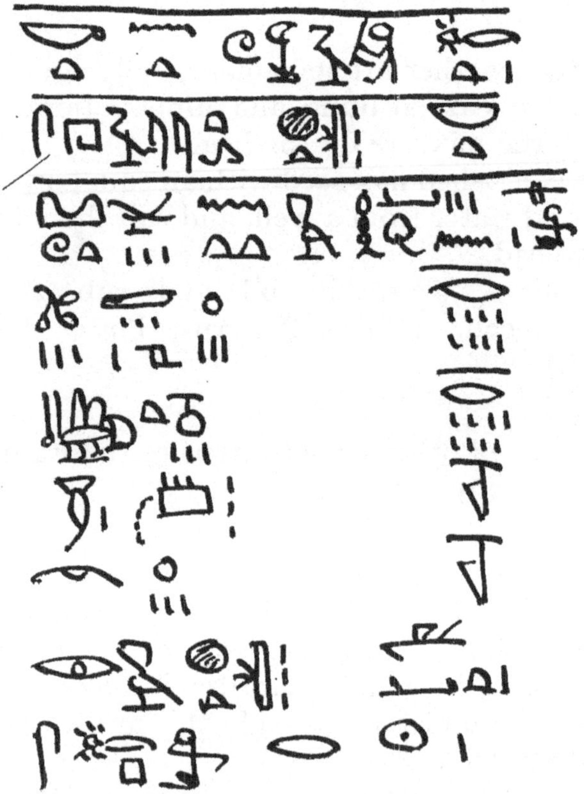

4. To STOP SUFFUSION OF BLOOD IN THE EYES. Take two shells of clay. Fill one of them with the powder of the fruit of the *dūm* palm [mixed with] the milk of a woman who hath given birth to a boy, and fill the other with cow's milk and keep it from curdling. In the morning fill both thine eyes with the mixture of *dūm* palm powder and woman's milk, and after that wash both eyes in the cow's milk four times a day for six days. (Ebers Papyrus, Plate LX.)

The following is a transcript of the hieratic text in hieroglyphs :

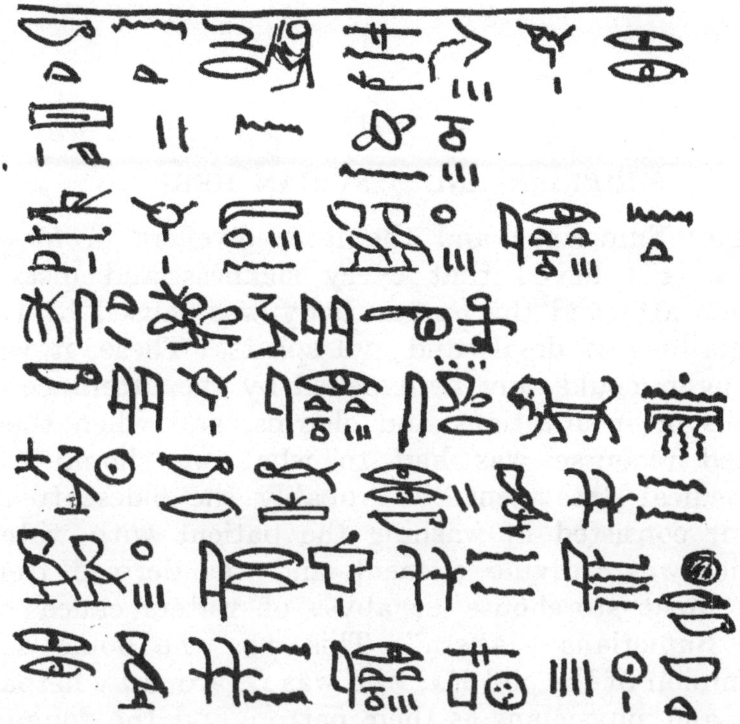

VII

SUMERIAN AND ASSYRIAN HERBALS

THE Sumerians and the later dwellers in Mesopotamia believed that every sickness and disease which attacked the human body was caused by the operations of devils and evil spirits. These, it was thought, could only be expelled by the utterance of spells or incantations and charms, and when these failed recourse was had to what we should call "medical treatment." Probably the oldest treatment consisted in washing the patient with water, which was a divine element, and was derived from the great storehouse or abyss of waters called by the Sumerians "APSŪ." This was the home and dominion of the god EA, who was regarded by herbalists and physicians as their patron, and the founder of the art of healing. At a later period many other gods were believed to be physicians, *e.g.* the goddess NINKHURSAG, and her company of eight gods, each of whom presided over one of the branches of medicine, and Ninazu, the "lord of physicians," or the Master-physician. The god NINURTA was credited with the power to destroy and render ineffective the spells of sorcerers and others, and his wife GULA used her great power in revivifying the dead.

When the Sumerians began to compile their Herbal cannot be said, but a tablet which was at one time in the Library of Ashurbanipal, King of Assyria, B.C. 668–626, at Nineveh, and is now in the British Museum (K 4023), has a note at the end of it which says that it was copied from a tablet which had been written in the second year of the reign of Enlil-bani, King of Isin, about B.C. 2201–2177. And the note refers to a tradition from the time of "the ancient rulers before the Flood which was in Shurippak." Thus it is clear that the Sumerian Herbal was in existence in the second half of the third millennium B.C. Copies of medical tablets have been found at "the city of Ashur" which are several centuries older than those of Nineveh, and the medical tablets discovered at Bogaz Koï prove that the Hittites possessed copies of texts which were probably made from Sumerian or Akkadian (Babylonian) archetypes. Whether the Sumerians were the discoverers of the arts of healing which they employed cannot be said. Their arts have much in common with those employed by the Egyptians, if we may judge by the contents of the Ebers Papyrus, and it seems as if the art of medicine had already become nationalized in the third millennium B.C. At all events it cannot be said with certainty that the Egyptians borrowed from the Sumerians, or that the Sumerians borrowed from the Egyptians; the probability is that both nations borrowed from a common source, and the present writer thinks that that source was far more likely to have been Asiatic than African. Of the folk-medicine of the aboriginal inhabitants of Mesopotamia, and that of the aboriginal inhabitants of Egypt, nothing whatever is known, but it is quite certain that few, if any, of the Egyptian and Sumerian herbalists and physicians ever succeeded in freeing themselves from the trammels of influence of magic and sorcery.

The knowledge which we possess of the Assyrian Herbal is derived from the baked clay tablets and fragments which have been found among the ruins of the great Library of the temples at Nineveh and the Royal Library of Ashurbanipal, King of Assyria, B.C. 668–626, at Nineveh. This king was a great patron of learning and he spared no pains in filling his Library with series of well-made, well-baked, and carefully written clay tablets dealing with grammar, history, religious and profane literature, magic, omens, incantations, divination, astrology, etc. Many of his tablets were written in two languages, Sumerian and Assyrian, and the information derived from them is practically the foundation of the modern science of Assyriology. Had these tablets come down to us in a complete state we should have been able to translate the medical texts and reconstruct the Assyrian Herbal without difficulty, but, alas, the number of complete tablets which Fate has saved from the Libraries of Nineveh are comparatively few, whilst the fragments of tablets number about 40,000! These all have been brought from Nineveh by the late Sir Henry Layard and the other excavators, who have been sent out by the Trustees, and they are now preserved in the British Museum. The condition of these fragments tells the story of the ill-treatment which they received on those awful days in the year 612 B.C. when Nineveh was captured by her enemies, and her palaces and temples were pillaged and burnt, and her precious literary treasures were smashed in pieces and their fragments scattered in all directions.

The scribes of Ashurbanipal compiled bilingual lists

of stars, countries, cities and towns, stones, animals, woods, trees, etc., and their lists of plants formed the various sections of the Assyrian Herbal, that is to say, the Herbal which was compiled in Assyria, probably in the seventh century B.C. The first to publish any portions of these lists was Sir Henry Rawlinson (see *Cuneiform Inscriptions of Western Asia*, Vol. II, London, 1866). Many scholars, English, French and German, began to give their attention to the medical texts generally, and to publish small groups of texts together with such translations as the knowledge available at the time permitted. Many scholars, *e.g.* Küchler, Scheil, Jastrow, Langdon, Virolleaud, Boissier and Ebeling, have made valuable contributions to the science of Mesopotamian medicine generally, but we owe such knowledge as we possess of the Assyrian Herbal entirely to Dr. Campbell Thompson, Fellow of Merton College, Oxford. Whilst serving in the British Museum he enjoyed ready access to the many thousand tablets and fragments of tablets of the great Nineveh (Kuyunjik) Collection, and made the large and valuable series of Lists of Assyrian Plants which were published in *Cuneiform Texts*, Vol. XIV, London, 1902. The texts there given are entirely distinct from the medical texts published by him in Vol. XXIII of the same work.

Between 1902 and 1920 various scholars published many fragmentary texts, with translations, but the results were wholly unsatisfactory, for they either left the vegetable medicines and drugs unidentified or translated the names of them haphazard. Thompson was the first to see that no real progress had been or could be made until the whole of the fragments of herbals and medical texts in the British Museum and elsewhere had been examined and published. Duplicates must be recognized and sorted out, and all the fragments which belonged together rejoined. To this great work he devoted himself, and his *Assyrian Herbal*, or monograph on Assyrian vegetable drugs, appeared in London in 1924. His study was based upon the texts of 120 cuneiform fragments published by Rawlinson or by himself in the official editions of the British Museum, and on the copies of 660 medical tablets published in his *Assyrian Medical Texts*, Oxford, 1923, and on previous publications of medical texts.

As a result of his studies we now know that the vegetable drugs known to the Assyrians were about 250 in number. The mineral drugs were about 120, and other drugs, still unidentified, were about 180 in number. To these must be added alcohols, fats, oils, honey, wax, and various kinds of milk (*Assyrian Herbal*, p. v). A list of all the drugs at present identified is given on pp. vii–xi. An examination of the plant lists of the Herbal shows that the ancient botanists adhered *in the main* to a definite arrangement. The herbalist had sufficient knowledge to classify plants according to his needs, but he does not arrange his plants in the order of modern botanists. He begins with grasses, and then follows with rushes and Euphorbiaceæ, reasonably enough, but he groups the Papaveraceæ and Cucurbitaceæ with other orders because the names for the principal plants begin with a certain cuneiform sign. He scatters Compositæ throughout his series. Thompson says: "The more the subject is studied, the more obvious appears to have been the great knowledge possessed by the doctors and chemists of Nineveh." When the *Assyrian*

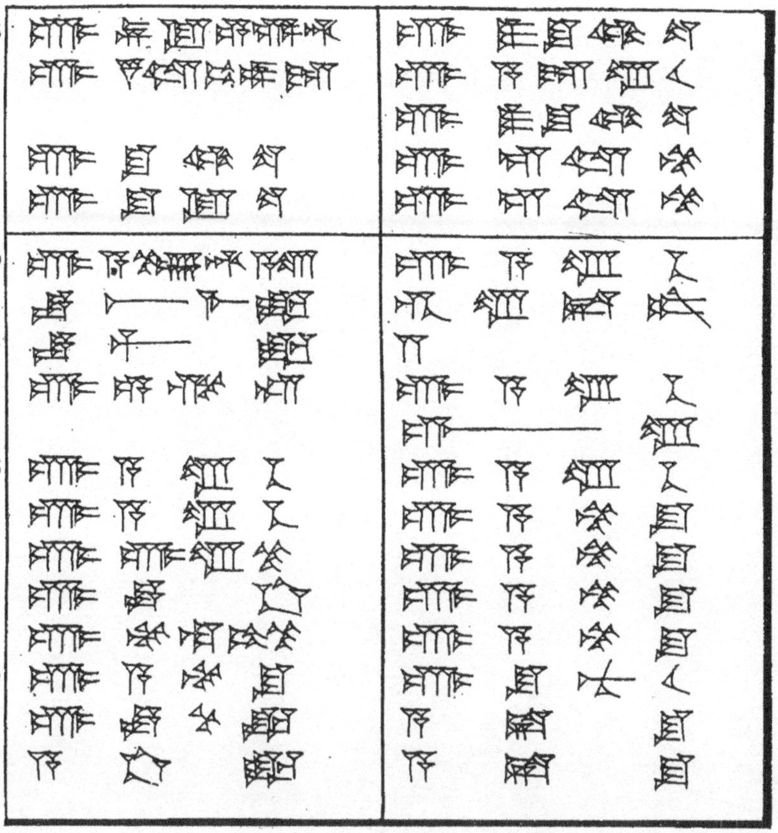

SECTION OF THE ASSYRIAN HERBAL FROM THE LIBRARY OF ASHURBANIPAL, KING OF ASSYRIA, AT NINEVEH.

(From the reverse of Brit. Mus. Tablet No. 4345, published by Dr. Thompson in *Cuneiform Texts*, Part XIV, Plate 28, and in his *Assyrian Herbal*, p. 21.)

Herbal was complete it contained the names of between 900 and 1000 plants, but the fragments now made available in their entirety show that many of these were synonyms. Thompson has in a great measure reconstructed the Assyrian Herbal, and, following each section of the text, he gives notes in which he discusses the names, colours and forms of the plants, and states what he believes to be their medicinal properties. He shows that the names by which we know many of the plants are derived from Sumerians through the Greek and Arabic languages, and among such may be mentioned apricot, asafœtida, saffron, liquidambar, galbanum, colocynth, carob, cardamom, cummin, opoponax, turmeric, cherry, flax, nard, silphium, phaseolus, myrrh, mulberry, mandrake, almond, poppy, styrax, sesame, cypress, lupin, etc.

Here may be given an extract from the great Assyrian Herbal from a tablet (K 4345) in the British Museum; in Thompson's reconstruction the lines are numbered 445–462. It will be noticed that nearly all the lines in both columns begin with the sign "u," which is read "sham," and indicates that what follows it is the name of a plant or of something made from a plant. The left-hand column of such lists often contains both the Sumerian ideographs for the plants, and Semitic names and synonyms and the right Semitic names. A transliteration of the first five lines of the extract will make this clear.

445	u ZAL.LU e-rish-ti	u ash-shu-ul-tu
446	u SHA.LAM.BI.TUR.RA	u a-ra-ru-u
447		u ash-shu-ul-tu
448	u shu-ul-tu	u si-lam-mu
449	u shu-lu-tu	u si-lam-mu.

As specimens of the Assyrian medical texts may be quoted :—

1. [If a man's eyes] are full of . . . . . thou shalt mix *Lolium* (and) flour of parched corn in beer and bind on; for three days to his eyes thou [shalt do this], renewing (it) thrice daily; on the fourth day thou shalt surround his eyes with *suadu* (and) opium, water in . . . . of clay and once, twice, or thrice his eyes thou shalt press: marrow of gazelle-bone to his eye[s thou shalt apply]. Then in opium thou shalt bray antimony (and) apply it to his eyes; thou shalt bray gall apples (and) apply dry to his eyes. Thrice daily thou shalt renew (it); thou shalt mix a paste of *mazi* (?), *barhush* (*N*. tamarisk), seed of *Kutru*, ... parched corn, *Lolium*; apply it dry to his head, bind his head, and for [three] days [do not take off]. On the fourth day thou shalt take it off and shave his head: apply thy paste to his eyes, [and he shall recover]. [Thompson, *Proc. Roy. Soc. of Medicine*, Vol. XIX, No. 3, p. 48.]

2. Incantation for toothache, which was believed to be caused by a worm gnawing at the root of the tooth :—

After Anu made the heavens, the heavens made the earth, the earth made the rivers, the rivers made the canals, the canals made the marsh, the marsh made the Worm. The Worm came weeping to Shamash, came unto Ea, her tears flowing: "What wilt thou give me for my food, what wilt thou give me to destroy?" "I will give thee dried figs and apricots." "Forsooth, what are these dried figs to me, or apricots? Set me amid the teeth, and let me dwell in the gums, that I may destroy the blood of the teeth,

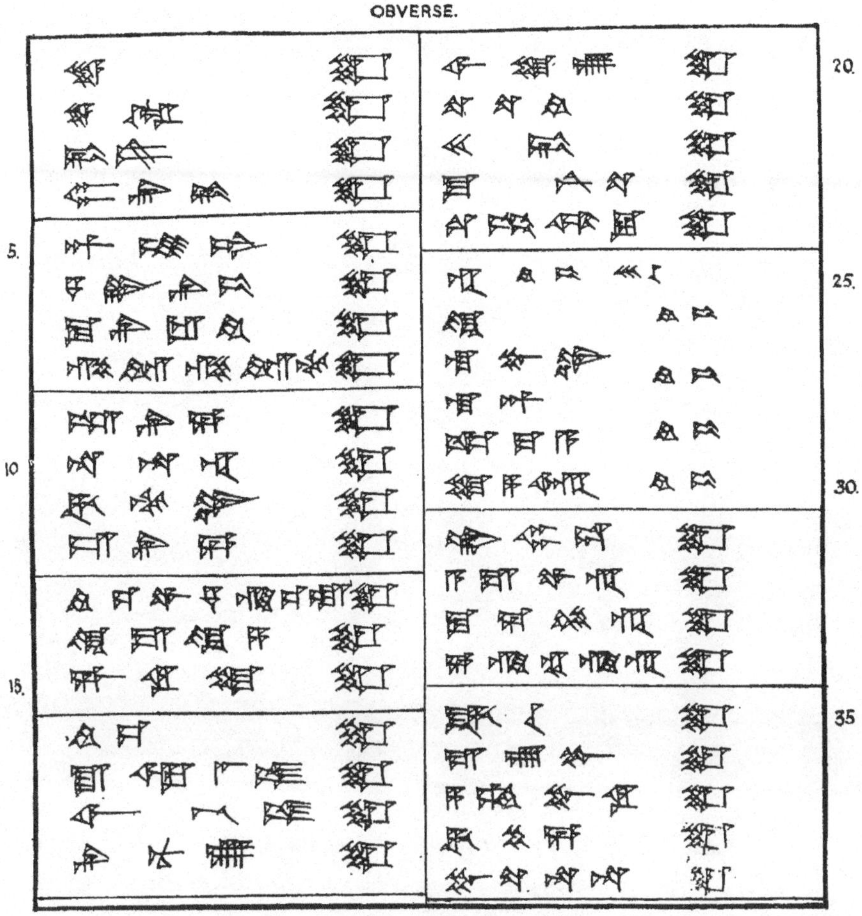

List of Plants in the Herb-garden of Merodach-Baladan II, King of Babylon, Cols. I and II.

(From Brit. Mus. Tablet No. 46226, published in *Cuneiform Texts*, Part XIV, Plate 50.)

REVERSE.

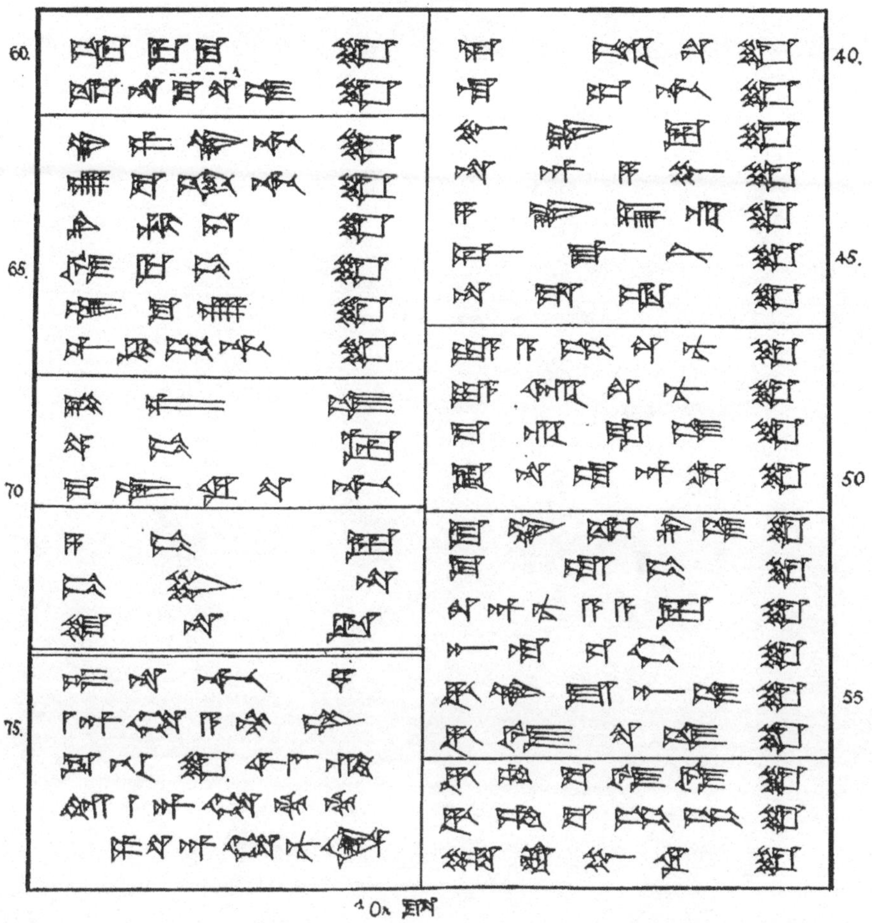

LIST OF PLANTS IN THE HERB-GARDEN OF MERODACH-BALADAN II, KING OF BABYLON, COLS. III AND IV.

(From Brit. Mus. Tablet No. 46226, published in *Cuneiform Texts*, Part XIV, Plate 50.)

and of the gums chew their marrow. So shall I hold the latch of the door." "Since thou hast said this, O Worm, may Ea smite thee with his mighty fist"! [*Ibid.*, p. 59.]

The Assyrian Herbal makes it quite clear that those who compiled it possessed a very considerable knowledge of herbs and plants and their properties, and we must assume that they took steps to ensure that a regular supply of medicinal plants should be forthcoming. This could best be done by establishing "physic gardens" in connection with the temples or the King's palace. Whether they did this or not cannot be said with certainty, but when we consider the great importance of herbs and plants in the Mesopotamian system of medicine, it seems very probable that they did. Now there is preserved in the British Museum a small clay tablet (No. 46226) which is inscribed in the neo-Babylonian character with a list of the plants which were in the garden of Merodach-Baladan II, King of Babylon, B.C. 721–710 and 703–702. It gives the names of 73 "garden-plants," arranged in groups in two columns. The sign which comes at the end of nearly every line indicates that the plants were strong-smelling (the onion is mentioned!), or that they emitted pleasant aromatic odours. This list was made for or by one Marduk-shumiddin, who describes himself as a worshipper of Marduk, from an older copy which, judging from the remark repeated in small characters in lines 25–30, was illegible in places. The docket gives the name of "Marduk-apal-iddina, the King," and the following line states that the copy was "written, revised, and correct according to its original." It might not be strictly accurate to say that the tablet gave a list of the contents of Merodach-Baladan's "Physic Garden," but there is no doubt that among the plants mentioned in the list are many that were used in medicine. Where the garden was situated cannot be said, but it was probably on the west bank of the Euphrates near the town of Hillah.

The great King of Assyria, Sennacherib, B.C. 705–681, also laid out gardens and parks round about Nineveh. On one of his inscribed prisms in the British Museum (No. 103,000) he says: "I laid out gardens above and below the city. I planted for my subjects, products of the mountains and of all countries, all the herbs of the land of Khatti, and murru plants, which flourished more than in their own country, all kinds of mountain vines, all kinds of foreign fruit trees, herbs and *sirdu* trees for my subjects." And this King seems to have introduced the cotton tree into Nineveh, for he says: "They clipped the trees that bore wool, and they shredded it for clothing."

Among the plants known to the Assyrians was one which appears in the famous Epic of Gilgamish; it was called "Shību issahir amelu," *i.e.* "the old man becometh young [again]." The immortal Uta-Napishtim told Gilgamish that it grew at the bottom of the sea, and that it would confer upon him immortality. Gilgamish weighted himself with stones, and let himself down on to the bed of the sea through an opening in the floor of his boat. He found the plant, plucked it, and ascended into his boat with it. Whilst he was on his way back to Erech, Gilgamish saw a pool of cold water, and setting the plant down he dived into the water and bathed. Whilst he was doing this a serpent discovered the whereabouts of the plant through its smell and ate it up! Thus Gilgamish lost his last chance of becoming immortal.

Thanks to the magico-medical texts which have been published in recent years it is now possible to describe the method of treatment employed by the Babylonian and Assyrian herbalist and physician. When a man fell sick in his house, sooner or later a messenger was sent to "fetch the doctor" from the temple. The Asu, or doctor, no doubt questioned the messenger fully, and when he had learned from him details concerning the sick man, he took his medical box and stocked it with the drugs, and perhaps instruments, such as a knife and a tube, which he thought would be required by him. Then with his staff or rod of office in his hand, and his box, he set out to go to the house of the sick man. But he did not go alone. He took with him a priestly official, whose title was "Ashipu," and who was learned in exorcisms, spells and incantations, and another official who was known as the "Bāru" or Seer. This last was skilled in the knowledge of omens.

As the three men made their way to the house of the sick man, the Bāru watched every person, animal or thing which they met, and proceeded to deduce omens from what he saw. He told the Ashipu what the omens portended, and this man began to recite the incantations which he thought would avert evil from the sick man. When the trio reached the house and went into the room of the sick man, the Asu examined him carefully and made his diagnosis, and meanwhile the Bāru continued to deduce omens from the state of the various members of the patient's body, whether his head was hot, or cold, or moist, whether there was foam on his lips, whether he was lying on his right or left side, or on his back, etc. As he told the Ashipu what such things portended, this official recited the incantations that were suitable. Meanwhile the Asu had decided what medicines were to be used, and when he had made them ready and began to administer them, the Ashipu continued to recite the incantations which were to drive out of the patient's body the devils or evil spirits that were the causes of his sickness. Thus medicine and magic went hand in hand, but any good effect which the medicines might produce was ascribed to the magical power of the incantations, and to the wisdom of the Bāru, who had read the omens rightly. In cases of prolonged illness the patient was removed to the temple, where a special chamber called the Kummu was provided for the reception of the sick, but the relatives of a patient were held to be responsible for his maintenance. Here in the Kummu chamber magical rites and ceremonies for the benefit of the sick were carried out in great detail. Magical signs and symbols and names were written on the walls, and series of prophylactic figures were employed to protect both the patient and the chamber from the attacks of devils. These figures were placed in boxes of burnt brick underneath the pavement, and the boxes were lined up against the walls, the open side of each box facing towards the centre of the chamber, the figures thus being on guard, as it were, over the living space. The figures were all of unbaked clay. Some of them had human bodies with birds' heads and wings, some of them were of males, and if nude were generally ithyphallic, or wholly obscene, and cat-headed figures, and figures of snakes, dragons, etc., were also found at Ur.

Incantations were recited over these figures, magical names were written on their hips, and a certain group of seven of them represented the seven Apkallu, or sages who lived before the Flood, and were the first to teach men incantations against sickness. Mr. Sidney Smith of the British Museum has discovered the ritual texts which deal with the prophylactic figures, and he has published translations of them, with notes, in a valuable paper on the figures actually found at Ur by Mr. C. L. Woolley in *Journal Royal Asiatic Society*, October 1926, p. 689 ff.

VIII

THE GREEK HERBALS

In the preceding pages the history of the Herbal in Egypt and Mesopotamia has been traced from the beginning of the third millennium B.C. to the reign of Ashurbanipal, King of Assyria, B.C. 681–668. It has also been shown that the system of medicine in use in those countries had much in common, and that the herbalists and physicians in both countries believed that both their craft and their medicines were of divine origin. Of the history of the Herbal after the Fall of Nineveh, which we now know (thanks to Mr. C. J. Gadd) took place B.C. 612, nothing is known, but there is little doubt that the medicines used in Egypt became known in Nubia and Northern Ethiopia and to the peoples of the Mediterranean, and those used in Babylonia and Assyria found their way into Persia, Armenia, Syria and Palestine. Throughout all these countries the belief that sickness and disease were caused by devils and evil spirits was general.

The Hellenes (Greeks), like the Sumerians and Egyptians, believed that the gods were the first herbalists and physicians, and that the art of healing was taught to man by them. Their first great god of medicine was Asklēpios or Æsculapius, the son of Apollo and the virgin Coronis. He was born in Epidaurus, and is said to have flourished about B.C. 1250. He learned his art from Cheiron, and was so successful in healing disease, and in raising the dead, that Zeus became jealous of him and slew him with a thunderbolt. He and his sons Machaon and Podalirius are mentioned by Homer (*Iliad*, ii. 731). He carried a staff, with a serpent, the symbol of renewed life, coiled round it. Hygieia, the goddess of health, was his daughter. He was worshipped in Rome under the form of a snake at the beginning of the third century B.C. There was never any suggestion that he wrote books of medicine. An ancient tradition says that Æsculapius was a native of Memphis in Egypt who emigrated to Greece, and that he introduced the knowledge of medicine into that country. Another legend says that when administering medicines or using the knife he recited incantations in order to make his drugs more effective.

But the real founders of Greek medicine and the compilers of the Greek Herbals were not the priests of Æsculapius, but the lay herb-doctors and physicians who were called "Asclepiadæ." Like the wandering "Hakîm" who is met with in towns and villages in Mesopotamia and the neighbouring countries at the present day, the Asclepiadæ earned their living by wandering about from place to place, and healing the sick folk wheresoever they found them. It is interesting to find a woman among the recognized herbalists of this early period, for Agamēde, daughter of Augeias, and wife of Mulius, was famed for her knowledge of the healing powers of all the plants that grow upon the earth. She is mentioned by Homer (*Iliad*, xi. 739). Homer also mentions the Egyptian queen Polydamna (*Odys.*, iv. 238), who gave Helen a drug (opium?) which would soothe every grief and abate anger.

The founders of many of the great Greek Schools of Medicine owed their learning in a great measure to the Egyptians. THALES of Miletus (B.C. 639–544), the founder of the Ionic School, was a pupil of Egyptian priests. PYTHAGORAS of Samos (B.C. 580–489), the founder of the School of Crotona, was a pupil of Un-nefer, a priest of Heliopolis. HIPPOCRATES (B.C. 460–377) of Cos, the "Father of Medicine," the second of this name in a family of very distinguished men, and the founder of a system of scientific medicine, derived a great deal of his learning from the Egyptians. He was the son of the Asclepiad Heraklides, who was the seventeenth in descent from Æsculapius, by the midwife Phaenarete, who was eighteenth in descent from Hercules. He was the first to banish magic and superstition from medicine, though even during his lifetime many practitioners, whilst using his remedies, resorted to magic and incantations to give greater effect to them. The drugs which he used—between 300 and 400 have been enumerated—were chiefly vegetable in character, but he employed copper, alum and lead in his medicines, and even common articles of food. There is no evidence that he compiled a Herbal, and therefore he most probably used the lists of plants which were known to Thales and Pythagoras when in Egypt.

The first Greek Herbal of which we have any mention consisted of lists of plants and their habitats, with short statements concerning their medicinal properties. This was compiled by DIOCLES CARYSTIUS, who was born at Carystus in Eubœa, probably in the first half of the fourth century B.C. He belonged to the Dogmatic School of Medicine which was founded by Thessalus (B.C. 380), Draco the physician and others. His Herbal is no longer extant, and of most of his other works only the names are known.

The great philosopher ARISTOTLE, the "Stagirite" (B.C. 384–322), the son of Nicomachus (a descendant of Machaon, a son of Æsculapius) by his wife Phæstis, was thought to have compiled the list of over 500 plants (*De Plantis*) which is usually included with his works, but modern critics attribute the list to a later writer, perhaps Theophrastus of Eresus.

THEOPHRASTUS (TYRTAMUS) was a native of Eresus in Lesbos; he was born about B.C. 372 and died in 285. He wrote two books on botany, and describes in his *Historia plantarum* over 500 plants; some of his statements are based on the knowledge of plants which he acquired at first hand during his travels, and others, especially those on foreign plants, from information supplied by caravan merchants. He may be regarded as the first scientific botanist, and his work contains parts of the OLDEST GREEK HERBAL known. For the text of the *Historia* see Wimmer's edition (Vratislaviæ, 1842) and Sir A. F. Hort's *Theophrastus: Enquiry into Plants*, London, 1916.

HEROPHILUS was a native of Chalcedon in Bithynia, and a prominent member of the Medical School of Alexandria; the dates of his birth and death are unknown, but he probably flourished in the first half of the third century B.C. He was severely criticized for administering large doses of vegetable compounds to his patients, and for the invention of heterogeneous mixtures of drugs. His work on plants, which is mentioned by Pliny (XXV. § 5), is no longer extant.

ANDREAS of Carystus, who was physician to Ptolemy IV. Philopator, wrote a work on plants, which is now lost; whilst in attendance on his master in his tent, Theodotus the Ætolian, who had hidden himself therein, killed him by mistake for the King (about B.C. 217).

NIGER (the Sextius Niger of Pliny) flourished about B.C. 30 and wrote a Herbal in Greek which is now lost.

CRATEUAS was a great herbalist and collector of plants, and physician to Mithridates VI. Eupator (B.C. 120–63) of Pontus, who was also a great herbalist, and famous for his skill in destroying people by poison. Crateuas wrote a Herbal in which he gave drawings of all the plants. Each drawing was preceded by the name of the plant and followed by a description of its use in medicine. He was the first to illustrate the Herbal. See Mr. C. Singer's article on the "Juliana Anicia Codex" at Vienna (written about A.D. 512), and the possible restoration of several of the drawings of Crateuas in *Journal Hellenic Studies*, Vol. XLVII. (1927), p. 4 ff.

All the Greek Herbals and medical works written between about B.C. 300 and B.C. 30 by the great botanists and herbalists of the School of Medicine of Alexandria were based upon the lists of plants and medical works of the Egyptians. The Sumerians and Egyptians made provision for receiving patients in their temples, and quarters for sick folk existed in the famous Museum at Alexandria. During the Ptolemaïc period a considerable amount of knowledge of Sumerian and Babylonian medicine must have found its way into Egypt, as a result of the campaigns of Alexander the Great in Western Asia in the fourth century B.C.

PAMPHILUS, a Greek herbalist who practised in Rome, wrote a Herbal in which the names of the

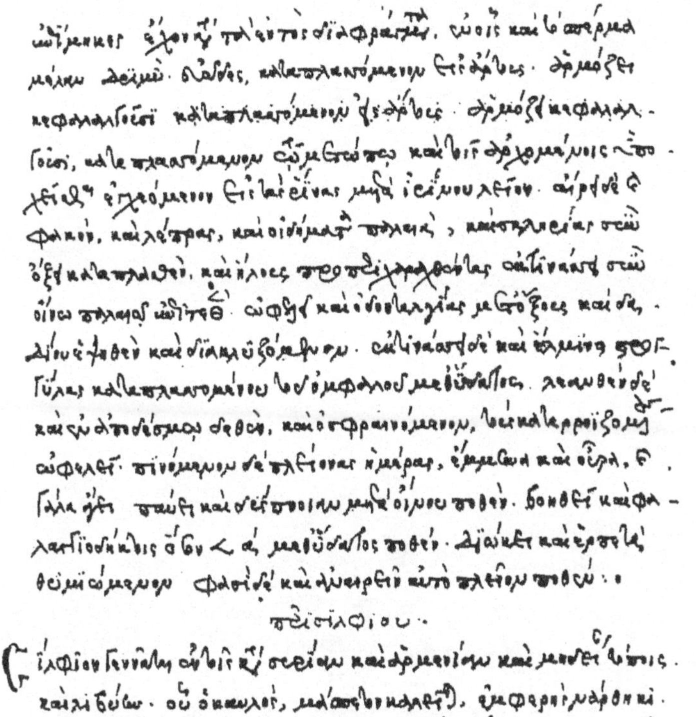

FACSIMILE OF A PAGE OF THE *De Materia Medica of* DIOSCORIDES, from a manuscript of the fifteenth century.

The lower half of the page contains a description of the *Silphiam* plant (*laserpitium*) and its uses as a food and a medicine.

(From Brit. Mus. Harl. MS. No. 5679, fol. 116*a*.)

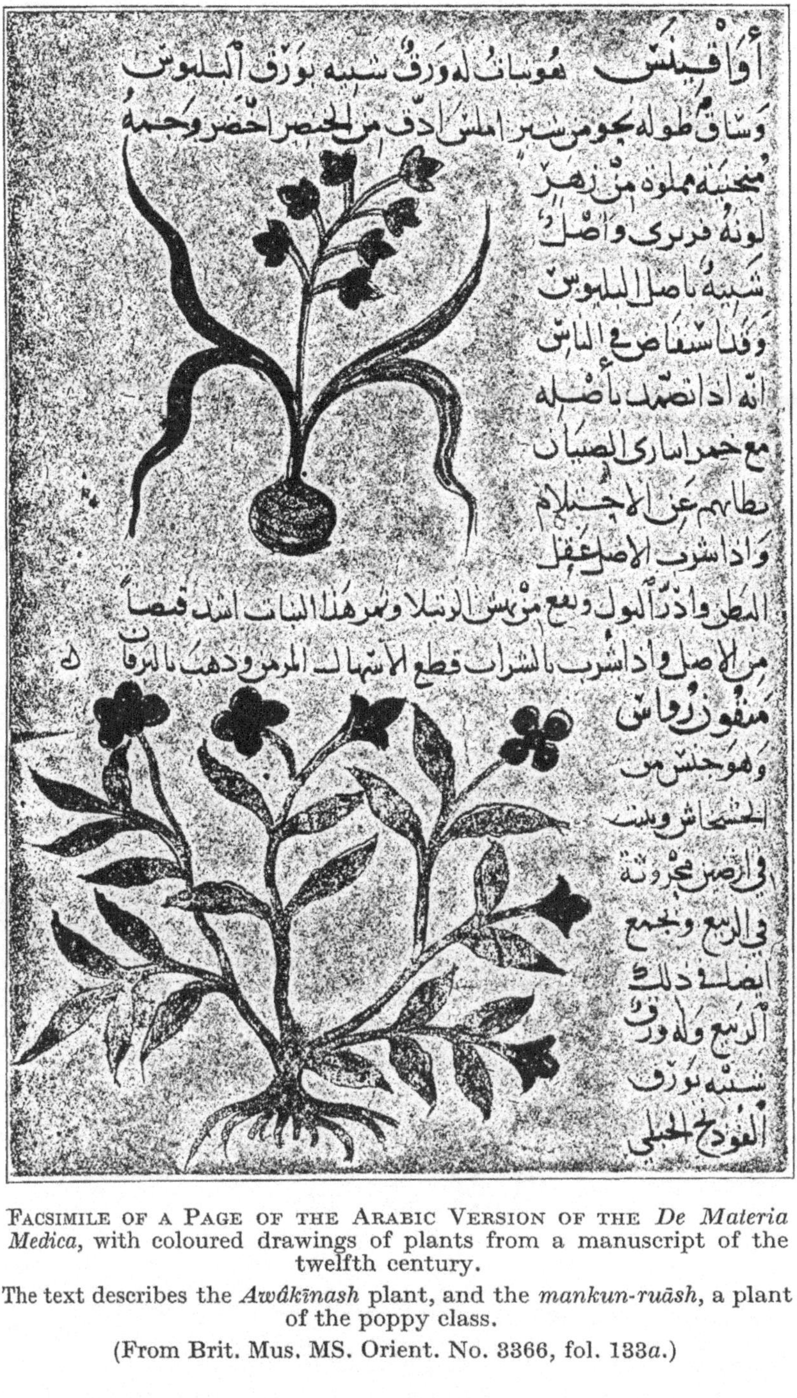

FACSIMILE OF A PAGE OF THE ARABIC VERSION OF THE *De Materia Medica*, with coloured drawings of plants from a manuscript of the twelfth century.

The text describes the *Awâkīnash* plant, and the *mankun-ruāsh*, a plant of the poppy class.

(From Brit. Mus. MS. Orient. No. 3366, fol. 133*a*.)

plants were arranged alphabetically; portions of it are preserved in the "Juliana Anicia Codex" mentioned above. Galen mentions Pamphilus, and accuses him of describing plants which he had never seen!

MENECRATES (Tiberius Claudius), physician to the Emperor Tiberius (A.D. 14–37), wrote a Herbal, which is lost. He was the inventor of *Diachylon plaster*.

We have now to consider the work of one of the greatest, if not the greatest, of the ancient herbalists, viz. PEDANIUS DIOSCORIDES (or Dioscurides), who was a native of Anazarba in Cilicia Campestris, and flourished in the early part of the second half of the first century of our era. He was one of the physicians attached to the Roman Army in Asia, and he collected a great deal of *general* information about plants at first hand. He owes his fame chiefly to his work *Περὶ ὕλης ἰατρικῆς*, which contains five books and is commonly known as *De Materia Medica*. The Greek text of this treatise has been published by Wellmann in the third volume of the collected works of the great herbalist (Berlin, 1914). A very useful summary of the results of recent study of the works of Dioscorides will be found in Singer, *Studies in the History and Method of Science*, Vol. II. p. 64, Oxford, 1921. Dioscorides travelled extensively in Greece, Italy, Germany, Gaul, Spain, etc., and as a result was able to discuss and describe about 400 plants. In his Herbal—that is to say, that portion of it which deals with plants—he gives the name of the plant and its Greek synonym, a description of it, its habitat and direction for its preparation as a medicine, and its medicinal effects. His Herbal is, in fact, a laborious compilation made from the works of Hippocrates,[1] Theophrastus of Eresus, Erasistratus, Andreas, Niger, Crateuas, Nikander and many other scientific botanists and herbalists. Among the drugs mentioned in his Pharmacopœia which are still to be found in the modern Pharmacopœias of Europe are :—almonds, aloes, ammoniacum, aniseed, belladonna, camomile, cardamoms, catechu, cinnamon, colchicum, colocynth, coriander, crocus, dill, galbanum, galls, gentian, ginger, hyoscyamus, juniper, lavender, linseed, liquorice, male fern, mallow, marjoram, mustard, myrrh, olive oil, pepper, peppermint, poppy, rhubarb, sesame, squill, starch, stavesacre, storax, stramonium, sugar, terebinth, thyme, tragacanth, wormwood. Two centuries later a number of synonyms were added to the Herbal of Dioscorides, and many figures of plants derived from illustrated Herbals, one being that of Crateuas. From this Recension of the Herbal of Dioscorides all the remaining manuscripts of the work have been copied, more or less completely from another Recension of the Herbal in which the synonyms were arranged alphabetically. ORIBASIUS of Pergamus (A.D. 325–403) based many portions of his works on it. This is not the place to trace the history of the transmission of the Herbal of Dioscorides from the fourth to the sixteenth century, which has been so admirably done by Mr. Singer in *Journal Hellenic Studies*, Vol. XLVII. p. 24 ff. It is sufficient to say that for more than thirteen centuries it was one of the principal text-books of herbalists and physicians throughout the civilized world.

The Greek Herbal assumed its final form in the

[1] About 130 of the plants known to Hippocrates are mentioned by Dioscorides.

hands of Claudius Galen, who was born at Pergamus in Moysia, about A.D. 130; he was the son of Nicon, an architect. He travelled extensively in Palestine and Asia Minor, and studied plants, and then set out to find the *gagates* stone, the use of which was believed to cure gout, epilepsy and hysteria. He wrote books on many subjects, and is said to have been the author of nearly 400 works! Of the 275 medical treatises attributed to him, 83 are genuine, 19 are doubtful and 48 are lost. About 83 of his works are extant, and of these some 80 exist only in manuscript. The most complete edition of Galen's works is that of Kühn in 22 volumes; a complete translation from the Greek of the entire works of Galen has never been made. Galen enjoyed great reputation as a philosopher and a medical teacher and law-giver. Throughout the whole Middle Ages this reputation continued undisputed, and, according to Baas, "by it he was the lord and master of medicine for fifteen hundred years." The Herbal of Galen is contained in Books VI–VIII of his work *Περὶ κράσεως καὶ δυνάμεως τῶν ἁπλῶν φαρμάκων*, which is commonly spoken of as *De Simplicibus*. These contain a list of drugs and their uses. A paragraph is given to each plant, and after its name come its synonym and its habitat; sometimes Galen gives a description of the plant itself, and he usually ends the paragraph with a statement as to its use in medicine.

Galen's work was so complete, and in a way so final, that no Greek or Roman botanist attempted to supersede the *De Simplicibus* by a work of his own. On the other hand, many herbalists based their treatises on plants on Galen's Herbal, and of them the most prominent was Oribasius of Pergamus

(A.D. 326–403). He was a pupil of ZENO at Alexandria, and became physician in ordinary to Julian the Apostate. But when he failed to heal the wound which his master received during the Persian campaign, he lost his position and his possessions. He wrote several works, and in his *Collecta Medicinalia*, or "Medical Compendium," he quotes not only well-known and famous writers like Hippocrates, Galen, Dioscorides and Diocles, but also lesser known botanists like Dieuches, Philumenus, Mnesistheus, etc. He was well acquainted with syphilis and gonorrhœa, and unceasingly proclaimed the value of dietetics and gymnastics.

IX

THE LATIN HERBALS

HERE must be mentioned two works which, though not Herbals in the true sense of the word, may be regarded as such, viz. the *De Re Rustica*, which in its earliest form was written by MARCIUS PORCIUS CATO CENSORINUS (B.C. 234–149), and the lengthy work on "Remedies derived from the Garden Plants" which fill Books XX–XXV of Pliny's *Natural History*. Cato's work contains a considerable number of native medical prescriptions of an old-fashioned character, and the magical spells or songs which were to be chanted whilst the medicines were being administered, *e.g.* "Huat, hanat, ista, pista, sista, damniato damnaustra." The following extract will give an idea of the character of Pliny's Herbal.

"CICHORIUM OR CHRESTON, OTHERWISE CALLED PANCRATION, OR AMBULA: 12 REMEDIES. Wild endive or cichorium has certain refreshing qualities used as an aliment. Applied by way of liniment, it disperses abscesses, and a decoction of it loosens the bowels. It is also very beneficial to the liver, kidneys and stomach. A decoction of it in vinegar has the effect of dispelling the pains of strangury; and, taken in honied wine, it is a cure for the jaundice, if unattended with fever. It is beneficial, also, to the bladder, and a decoction of it in water promotes the menstrual discharge to such an extent as to bring away the dead fœtus even. In addition to these qualities, the magicians state that persons who rub themselves with the juice of the entire plant, mixed with oil, are sure to find more favour with others, and to obtain with greater facility anything they may desire."

But the Italians of the third century after Christ were satisfied neither with their own native and simple prescriptions, nor the more scientific remedies of Dioscorides and Galen and works like the medical poem of Quintus Serenus Samonicus. The writer insisted on the value of magical formulas and the numbers 3, 7 and 9, and revived the amulet, which was derived from the Gnostics of the Basilidian sect, and is here given in its two principal forms. One or other of them was to be written on a piece of paper and folded in the form of a cross. The paper was to be hung round the neck by means of a cord made of a special kind of grass, and to lie on the naked flesh of the person who was suffering from any kind of fever for nine days. At midnight on the ninth day the patient was to rise up and go to a river or running stream, and at the first glimpse of dawn he was to throw the paper into the stream. The magic letters were supposed to draw the fever spirit into the paper, which the river would carry towards the rising sun that it might be burned up by his rays.

(1) ABRACADABRA
BRACADABR
RACADAB
ACADA
CAD
A

(2) ABRACADABRA
ABRACADABR
ABRACADAB
ABRACADA
ABRACAD
ABRACA
ABRAC
ABRA
ABR
AB
A

Towards the end of the fourth century A.D. Theodorus Priscianus, physician in ordinary to the

Emperor Gratian, wrote a Herbal, and Lucius Apuleius produced his *Herbarium* a little later. The *De Simplicibus* of Galen and the *De Materia Medica* of Dioscorides were translated from Greek into Latin at the end of the fifth or the beginning of the sixth century, and during the succeeding centuries various Recensions of them came into being, and short medical works by other writers were incorporated in them.

X

THE HERBAL IN SYRIAC

For nearly four centuries the Alexandrian School of Medicine (founded about B.C. 260) sent out into the countries round the Mediterranean scientific herbalists and botanists, skilled anatomists and wise and learned physicians. Alexander the Great had made Alexandria the greatest trading centre in the world, and the Ptolemies, his successors, made its Medical School to excel all others in learning. The discoveries made in Alexandria by the physicians who dissected the dead and vivisected the living in pursuit of the knowledge of the secrets of Nature were quickly made known to the Jewish physicians in Jerusalem and Damascus, and other cities on the great caravan roads leading towards the East. Little by little the knowledge of Greek medicine and the Herbals of Dioscorides and Galen became known in the literary cities of Āmid, or Diyarbakr, and Edessa, and before the close of the fifth century A.D. translations of Greek medical works began to be made into Syriac. This is proved by a statement of Bar Hebræus in his *Chronicle* (ed. Bruns and Kirsch, Leipzig, 1789, p. 62), which reads: "And Sapor (I., A.D. 240–273) built for himself a city which was like unto Constantinople, and its name was Gundhī Sābhōr (Bēth Lapāt), and he settled his Greek wife therein. And there came with her skilled men from among the Greek physicians,

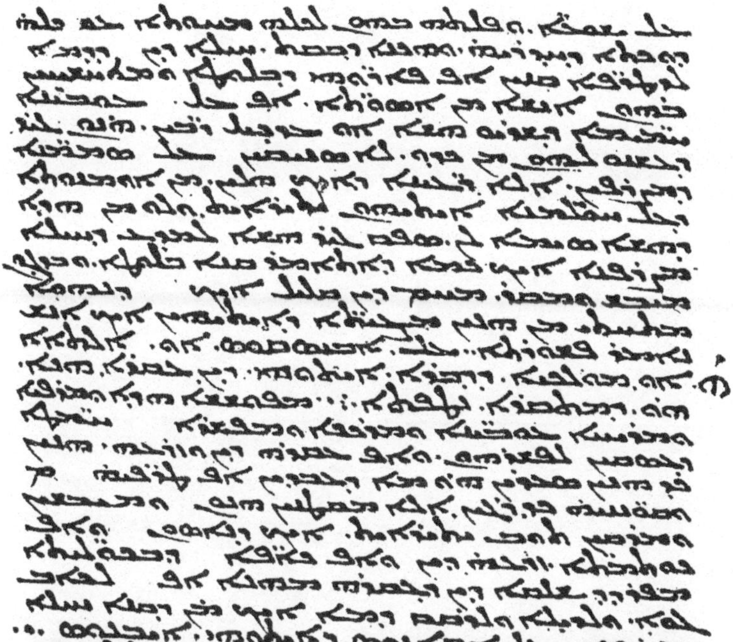

A Page from the Syriac Version of Galen's Herbal.

(From Brit. Mus. Add. No. 14661, fol. 25*a*.)

and they sowed the system of medicine of Hippocrates in the East. And there were also excellent Syrian physicians, such as Sargis (Sergius) of Rīsh Ainā, who was the first to translate the philosophical and medical works of the Greeks into Syriac . . . Gōsyōs (*i.e.* Gesius Petræus, who flourished in the reign of the Emperor Zeno) translated his book from Greek into Syriac." Bar Hebræus mentions several Syrians who wrote medical works in their native tongue. But most of their books are no longer extant. As to Sergius of Rīsh Ainā, we know that he was a good Greek scholar, and well versed in the philosophy of Aristotle; he was Archiater in his native town. The British Museum possesses copies of some of his translations from Galen's works, and in Add. 14661 we have a Syriac version of Books VI–VIII of his *De Simplicium Medicamentorum*, which may be regarded as a Syrian Herbal. This manuscript is one of the famous Nitrian Collection and was written in the sixth or seventh century: a reproduction of a page of it is here given. In the text Galen deals with the plant hibiscus (*Malva officinalis*), ābānōs, or ebony wood, and the olive tree.

In 1889 I found among the Nestorians at Mōsul an ancient manuscript of a great Syriac work called "Kethābhā dhe Sammānē," or "Book of Medicines." I was able to obtain a copy of this work, and it was subsequently published with an English translation by the Royal Society of Literature (see Budge, *Syrian Anatomy, Pathology and Therapeutics*, 2 vols., London, 1913). The first part of the book contains translations from the Greek, and is clearly based upon the writings of Dioscorides or Galen, in fact deals with medicine from the scientific point of view of the

Greeks. The second part includes a large number of native prescriptions, many of which were taken from the native medical works of the Babylonians and Assyrians, and curiously enough have much in common with the prescriptions given in the Ebers Papyrus. Spells and incantations were, of course, used freely.

The following are examples of the prescriptions in the Syriac "Book of Medicine."

1. *The* GREAT ANTĪRĀ *medicine, which is to be used for ailments of the throat, and which is to be blown into the mouth in the form of a dry powder.*

Take in equal quantities :

Crocus, Root of mountain rose, Ammoniac, Swallowwort, Pyrethrum, Peppercorns (long and round), Liquorice root, Purple balaustion, Rose (yellow) leaves, Glaucium, Phœniceum, Wood lettuce, Incense plant berries, Crocus root, Green gall nuts, Green myrobalanus chebula, Lycium, Glaucium, Persian *sathrē*, Pomegranate rind, Ferns, Aloes, Acacia, Indian salt, Daucus gingidum, Nard, Amomum, Ginger, Aniseed, Seed of rock parsley, Samterīn, Salsola, Cardamoms, Reed of incense plant, Lithargyrum, Arsenic, Krōkōmaghmā, Costus, Myrrh, Dog-excrement, Verdigris (?), Tamarix, Caryophyllus aromaticus, Vine mould, Seed of roses, Balsam bark and Cassia.

Pound all these well together, reduce them to a powder, and apply sometimes in the form of a powder, and sometimes mixed with honey in the form of a gargle.

2. *A medicine for gangrene in the mouth.*

Verdigris, Pyrethrum, Persian salt, 1 drachm each.

Ginger, Burnt peppercorns, Pilḍalpon, 2 drachms each.

Crush to a powder, dip thy finger in it and rub it on the teeth and gums. Then dip a strip of linen in vinegar, squeeze it dry, and dip it in the powder, and lay the strip on the place where the boils are.

XI

THE HERBAL IN ARABIC

THE pre-Muhammadan Arabs first became acquainted with the Greek Herbal and Greek medicine through the Jewish teachers of medicine who had studied at Alexandria, and the Syrian Christians of the famous School at Edessa. When the Nestorians became all-powerful in this School, the Government disbanded the pupils and closed it. It was reopened by Bishop Ibas in A.D. 435, but was finally dissolved by the Emperor Zeno in A.D. 489. The pupils fled to Nisibis, where Bar-Sāwma founded another School, which flourished for a considerable time. From the fifth century onwards the Syrians translated Greek medical works into Syriac, and from these translations the Arab physicians made translations into their own language. The most important of these were: GEORGE, the son of Bokht-Ishô, physician to Al-Mansûr the Khalīfah in the eighth century; GABRIEL, physician to Hārūn ar-Rashīd, who died at Baghdād A.D. 828; HONAIN IBN ISHĀK AL-IBĀDĪ, who translated from the Syriac the works of Hippocrates, Dioscorides, Galen, and Paul of Ægina, and died in 873. ISAAC, son of the last-named, and HOBAISH his nephew, translated many Greek works into Syriac and Arabic. According to Ibn Juljul, quoted by Abi Usaibiah, the work of Dioscorides on *Materia Medica* was translated from the Greek into Arabic by STEPHEN, son of Basil, a Christian Arab who flourished at Baghdād under the Khalīfah Mutawakkil, A.H. 240 (A.D. 853). Ibn Juljul says that Stephen gave the Arabic equivalent for the Greek name of the drug whenever he knew it, and when he did not he transcribed the Greek name into Arabic letters (De Sacy, *Relation de l'Égypte*, Paris, 1810, p. 495). The Brit. Mus. MS. Or. 3366 contains two of the five books of the work of Dioscorides (the third and the fourth), and attached to many of the descriptions of the plants are neat coloured drawings (see p. 61).

The greatest botanist produced by the Arabs in the Middle Ages was ABD-ALLĀH IBN AL-BAITĀR, who was born at Malaga, and died at Damascus A.H. 646 (A.D. 1248). He travelled extensively in Greece, Egypt and Asia Minor, and collected a vast amount of botanical knowledge at first hand. He was director of the Medical School of Cairo under Malik al-Kāmil (died 1237), and whilst there he compiled the great ARABIC HERBAL. He based his work on the Herbals of Theophrastus, Dioscorides and Galen, and his great knowledge enabled him to correct several mistakes in their works. His Herbal contains the names of nearly 800 plants, and he included in it the names of many Persian and Indian drugs (see the translation of J. von Sontheimer, 2 vols., Stuttgart, 1870–72).

Though the Arabs adopted with alacrity Greek medicine and Greek treatment of disease, they never gave up the use of charms and amulets and spells of all kinds. In the time of the Hijrah (June 20th, A.D. 622) they believed, and they still believe, that a few verses of the Kur'ān, if written on a paper which is steeped in a bowl of water, will turn the water into a most powerful medicine which will heal the sick believer, and bring disaster and even death upon the unbeliever. The man who carries an agate upon which the really beautiful "Ayāt al-Kursī" or "Throne-verse" is engraved, is considered to be protected from the attacks of wicked men, and from the assaults of vampires, and the Jinn, and spirits of the night, and the dead who are damned.

XII

COPTIC LISTS OF PLANTS

THE Copts, that is to say, the Egyptians who accepted the teaching of St. Mark in the first century of our era, and embraced Christianity, seem to have eschewed medical science as taught by the physicians of the famous School of Medicine of Alexandria, and to have been content with the methods of healing employed by their ancestors. No Coptic Book of Medicine has hitherto been discovered, and the oldest remains of their literature are wholly theological and patristic in character. Egypt was conquered by the Arabs A.D. 640, and Nubia twelve years later, and when the Arabs began the work of administering the country they found that the efforts of their governors and officers were hampered by their ignorance of the Coptic language, and the machinery of the Government was worked principally by Copts. In the ninth and tenth centuries the persecution of the Copts by the Arabs began, and for some three centuries the Christians in Egypt and Nubia and on the Island of Meroë suffered greatly. During this period Arab writers began to compose Grammars and Vocabularies of the Coptic language, and many of these are extant in modern manuscripts. (See Rieu, *Supplement to the Catalogue of Arabic MSS. in the British Museum*, No. 47, and Crum, *Catalogue of Coptic MSS.*, p. 384 ff.) In one of these (Brit. Mus. Orient. 1325) we have a copy of the "Scala Magna" of Abū al-Barakāt, commonly known as Ibn Kabr, who died A.D. 1363, and a facsimile of fol. 117*a* is given on p. 81. In one section we have a list of trees, a list of vegetables and plants possessing aromatic perfumes, and a list of seeds, both agricultural and medical—in fact, a kind of COPTIC HERBAL. The lists are bilingual, Coptic and Arabic. The following is a transcript of the Coptic names of plants which are given on p. 81.

1. BERSI, chrysalocanne, golden seed.
2. MIT, parsley (for garlands).
3. KRAM, carthamus silvestris.
4. SERINON, petrosclinum, rock parsley.
5. STAPINARI, pastinacea, daucus, parsnip, carrot.
6. AMISI, mentha gentilis.
7. AUS-ON, mentha montana.
8. AMIRON, arum (aron), wake-robin, cuckoo-pint.
9. BASHOUSH, ruta, rue.
10. EMTOTF, ruta montana, wild rue.
11. BETIKE (BETUKE?), wild apple, love apple, mandragora. The Arabic has the wild *bādingān*, *i.e.* the "egg-plant."
12. AL-MANTALŌPT, egg-plant, *bādingān*.
13. HTIT, holus, cabbage, beet, turnip, colewort.
14. SŌOUH EN KOUMARION, Arab. *bādingān*, egg-plant.
15. BUTIKE, Arab, wild egg-plant.
16. KOLOGINTHE, colocynth.
17. BENT EN TJLADJ, young gourd, pumpkin.
18. AGRIOLAKONON (*sic*), wild turnip (?).
19. KOLAKINON, Arab. *Al-aspānākh*, spinach.
20. MOLOKHIA, Arab. *malukhīyah*.
21. BAKINON, Arab. *bāmīya*.
22. ŌB, lactuca, lettuce.
23. EDJI, porrum.
24. KOGILĒ, turnip.
25. BERSHAU, coriander.
26. EXOMOU, eruca, colewort.
27. SAMNOKKHOS (?). . . . .
28. ANNOSHER, wild endive.
29. KEFRIOS, mountain rue.
30. KANON, garden rue.
31. SARIS, reed, chicory, asphodel.

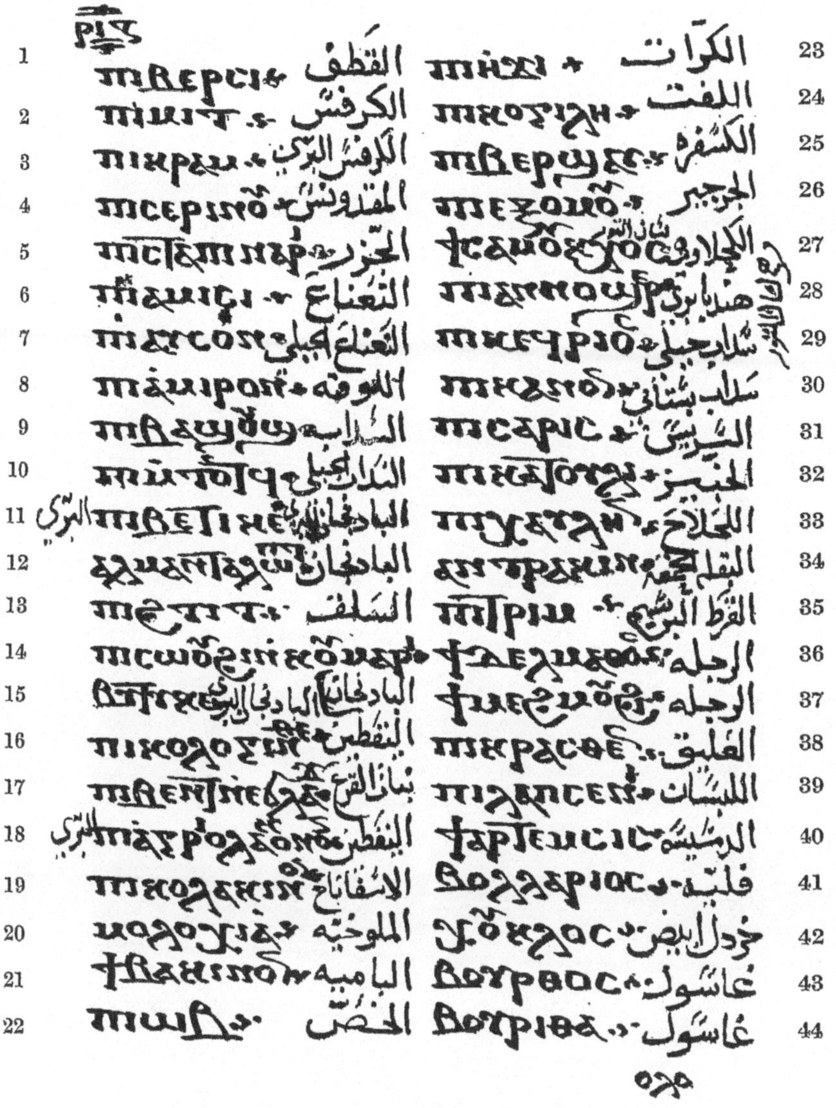

A Page from Ibn Kabr's List of Vegetables.
(From Brit. Mus. MS. Orient. No. 1325, fol. 117*a*.)

32. Katouli, mallows.
33. Khaulē. . . . .
34. Antrakin, vegetables in general.
35. Trim, trifolium. Arab. *bursīm*.
36. Delmathos, portulaca, purslain.
37. Mehmouh, portulaca, purslain.
38. Krasthec, blackberry.
39. Lapsen, Arab. *libsān*.
40. Artemsis, Artemisia abrotonum, southernwood.
41. Bollarios, an Indian (?) vegetable.
42. Khouklos, white mustard.
43. Bourthos, euphorbium spurge.
44. Bouritha, euphorbium spurge.

XIII

THE ETHIOPIAN (ABYSSINIAN) HERBAL

NOTHING is known of the means of healing sickness employed by the aboriginal Ethiopians, but we may assume that the "medicine men" of the day had a knowledge of the curative power of water, and were acquainted with the properties of certain plants, both helpful and harmful, and oils. It is possible that a limited knowledge of Egyptian medicine filtered into Ethiopia by way of Nubia, and that the Arabs from Yaman, who invaded the country from the sea about B.C. 1000, may have brought with them the system of medicine which was in use at that time in the neighbouring country of Babylonia. With the coming of the Greek merchants to Adulis and Aksūm in the first century of our era came some knowledge of the medical skill of the Alexandrian School, and this was greatly added to when the Ethiopians embraced Christianity about A.D. 350. But though the King and the great officials of his Court employed herb-doctors and physicians from the West, the people generally adhered to their beliefs in the native "medicine men," who relied absolutely on spells and charms to effect cures. Christians as well as pagans used spells, only for the names of demons and devils they substituted the names of the Persons of the Trinity, the Twelve Apostles, the Seven Archangels, the Four-and-Twenty Priests of heaven, etc.

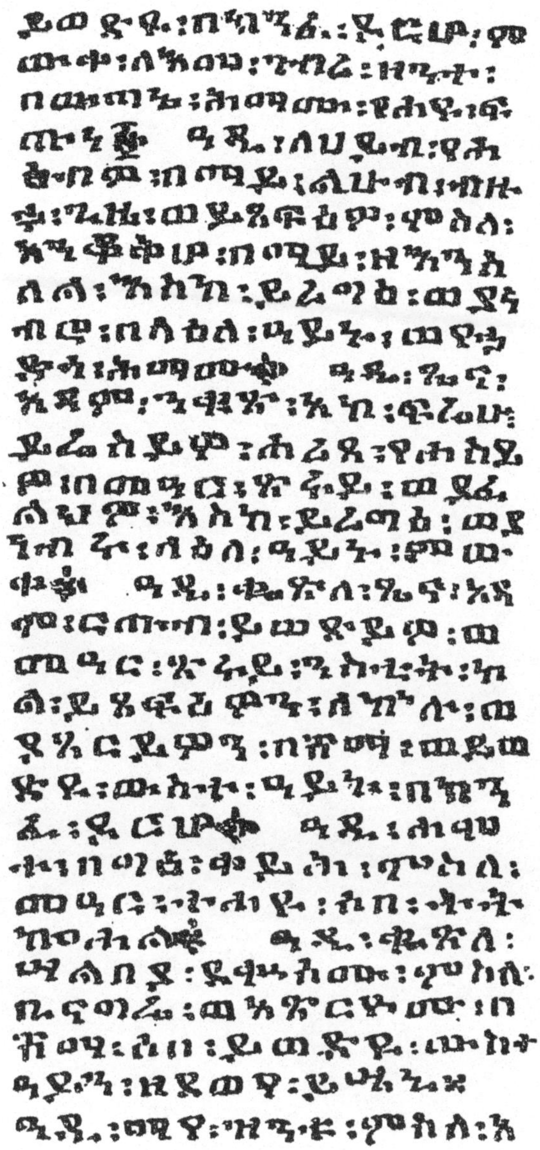

Facsimile of a Column from an Ethiopic Book of Medicine.

(From Brit. Mus. Add. 20741, fol. 4*b*.)

The native doctors who attended the sick in Ethiopia must, we should think, have had books containing copies of prescriptions in Ethiopic, but nothing of the kind has yet been discovered, except the MS. Add. 20741 now in the British Museum. This little book—it contains only 14 folios—is entitled "MAṢ-ḪAFA FAWES," and is described as a "Book of healing for every kind of sickness in all the members. They (*i.e.* the prescriptions) were collected by the ancient wise men so that they might be a means of relief for all the sick." The prescriptions in this book are of a very simple character, and many of them resemble the shorter prescriptions found in the Ebers Papyrus. The first of them deal with the head generally, and then follow receipts for medicines for individual members of the body, *e.g.* the eyes, the ears, the mouth, etc. Most of the sicknesses in Ethiopia are caused by exposure to the extremes of heat and cold, insufficient and improper food, and fevers of all kinds; epilepsy, St. Vitus's dance, dysentery, colic, diarrhœa, cholera, etc. have always been very general in the country. Among women miscarriages and sterility are common.

The British Museum also possesses a large Book of Medicine "MAṢḪAFA MADHANĪT" (Oriental 828) written in AMHARIC, that is to say, the modern language of Abyssinia, and in the title it is said that it went forth from Jerusalem. It is about a century old, and it belonged to Walda Gīyōrgīs Wasan Sagad, King of Shoa, who died in 1812. The actual prescriptions are very short, but many of them are accompanied by long spells and charms which resemble those of the prescriptions of Egypt and Babylonia and Assyria. The Christian in Ethiopia often relied for relief from his pain on pictures of the Virgin Mary and the Archangels Michael and Gabriel, and little crosses made of wood or bone which were held by him or laid on the suffering member or limb.

On p. 85 will be found a facsimile of a column of Ethiopic text from the manuscript Add. 20741, and it contains several prescriptions for rheum in the eyes, ophthalmia, blood in the eyes and defective sight generally. For inflammation, let him bathe the eyes with hot water for a long time. Then take extract of the scented *adām* plant, which has not flowered, and add thereto fine flour, and rub them down together into a paste, and lay it when moist on the eyes. Or, take the leaves of the scented *adām* plant, macerate them, add run honey, and a little apple, make them all into a firm paste, and dry the eyes, and apply the mixture to them with the feather of a cock. Or, take the gall of a red lamb (or sheep), and honey, and the patient will find relief if his eyes be smeared with [the mixture]. Or, take the fronds of the *shalbayā* plant, and pound them up with acid (*bīnāgrē* = vinegar), and dry them with a cloth. When these are laid upon the eyes of the sick man he will recover.

The difficulty of translating the prescriptions in both the Ethiopic and Amharic Book of Medicine is great, because it is well-nigh impossible to identify the drugs. The first in modern times to study the botany of Abyssinia was James Bruce, who in his *Travels*, Vol. VII, London, 1805, p. 117 ff., describes a number of the most important trees and plants in that country. It was he who made known to European scholars the Wāgīnōs plant (*Brucea antidysenterica*), the bark of which is such a wonderful specific

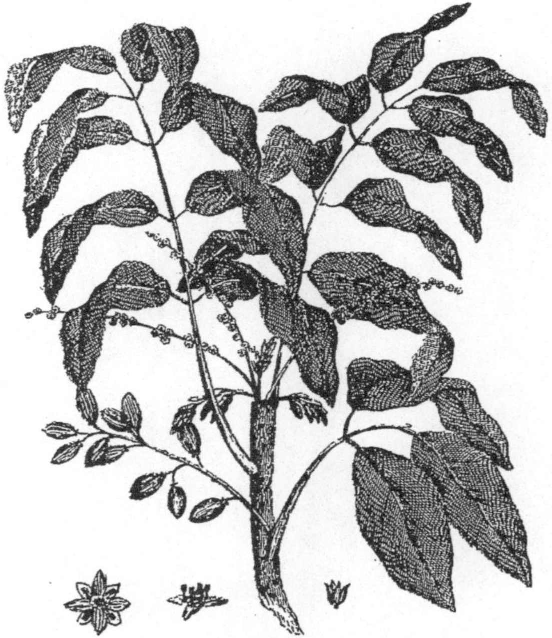

THE WĀGĪNŌS PLANT
(*Brucea antidysenterica*).

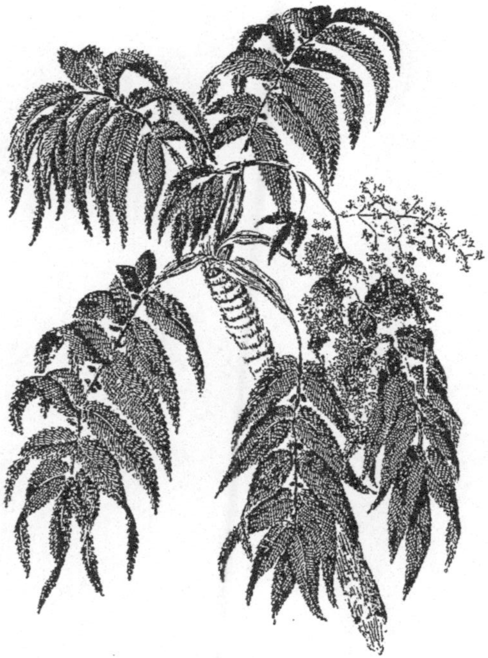

THE KUSSŌ TREE
(*Bankesia Abyssinica*).

for dysentery, and the Kussō (*Bankesia Abyssinica*), the flowers of which, being steeped in water, produce a liquid which is taken by almost every native in order to expel worms from the body. The figures of the plant and the tree given on p. 89 are reproduced from drawings by Bruce.

INDEX

More Books from Cornerstone

Simplified Scientific Astrology
by Max Heindel
6x9 Softcover 204 pages
ISBN 1613420749

Camp Cookery
by Horace Kephart
6x9 Softcover 170 pages
ISBN 1613420862

Initiation and its Results
by Rudolf Steiner
6x9 Softcover 134 pages
ISBN 1613420927

The Minor Prophets
by F. W. Farrar
6x9 Softcover 252 pages
ISBN 1613421079

Letters on Occult Meditation
by Alice A. Bailey
6x9 Softcover 372 pages
ISBN 1613420978

Angelic Wisdom:
Concerning the Divine Love and the Divine Wisdom
by Emanuel Swendenborg
6x9 Softcover 388 pages
ISBN 1613420889

Cornerstone Book Publishers
www.cornerstonepublishers.com

More Books from Cornerstone

More Books from Cornerstone

The Knights Templar and the Church
by Charles G. Addison
6x9 Softcover 236 pages
ISBN : 1-934935-22-0

History of the Secret Societies of the Army
by Charles Nodier
6x9 Softcover 260 pages
ISBN: 1-934935-24-7

New Orleans - The Place and the People
by Grace King
6x9 Softcover 426 pages
ISBN 1-613420-00-5

The Occult Life of Jesus of Nazareth
by Alexander Smyth
6x9 Softcover 326 pages
ISBN 1613420986

With the Adepts:
An Adventure Among the Rosicrucians
by Franz Hartmann
6x9 Softcover 124 pages
ISBN 1613420684

A Ghost of a Chance
by Evelyn Klebert
6x9 Softcover 96 pages
ISBN: 1-887560-50-5

More Books from Cornerstone

The Ancient Wisdom
by Annie Besant
6x9 Softcover 178 pages
ISBN: 1-934935-08-5

A Journey into Theosophy
by C.W. Leadbetter
6x9 Softcover 218 pages
ISBN: 1-887560-93-9

The Trial of Jeanne D'Arc
trans. by W.P. Barrett
Large Format, 8.5 x 11 Softcover 250 pages
ISBN: 1-934935-05-0

The Stone of the Philosophers
An Alchemical Handbook
Edited by Michael R. Poll
6x9 Softcover 368 pages
ISBN: 1-887560-85-8

An Esoteric Reading of Biblical Symbolism
by Harriet Tuttle Bartlett
6x9 Softcover 232 pages
ISBN 1613420803

Brother of the Third Degree
by Will L. Garver
6x9 Softcover 228 pages
ISBN: 1-887560-43-2

Cornerstone Book Publishers
www.cornerstonepublishers.com

Made in the USA
Monee, IL
08 November 2026

67382853R00069